S.Cary & Larry Borysyk

NUTRITION,
PHYSICAL FITNESS,
AND HEALTH

International Series on Sport Sciences

Series Editors: **Richard C. Nelson and Chauncey A. Morehouse**

The principal focus of this series is on reference works primarily from international congress and symposium proceedings. These should be of particular interest to researchers, clinicians, students, physical educators, and coaches involved in the growing field of sport science. The Series Editors are Professors Richard C. Nelson and Chauncey A. Morehouse of The Pennsylvania State University. The series includes the eight major divisions of sport science: biomechanics, history, medicine, pedagogy, philosophy, physiology, psychology, and sociology.

Each volume in the series is published in English but is written by authors of several countries. The series, therefore, is truly international in scope and because many of the authors normally publish their work in languages other than English, the series volumes are a resource for information often difficult if not impossible to obtain elsewhere. Organizers of international congresses in the sport sciences desiring detailed information concerning the use of this series for publication and distribution of official proceedings are requested to contact the Series Editors. Manuscripts prepared by several authors from various countries consisting of information of international interest will also be considered for publication.

The *International Series on Sport Sciences* serves not only as a valuable source of authoritative up-to-date information but also helps to foster better understanding among sport scientists on an international level. It provides an effective medium through which researchers, teachers, and coaches may develop better communications with individuals in countries throughout the world who have similar professional interests.

International Series
on Sport Sciences, Volume 7

NUTRITION, PHYSICAL FITNESS, AND HEALTH

Edited by:

Jana Pařízková, M.D., D. Sc.
Research Institute
Faculty of Physical Education
Charles University
Prague, Czechoslovakia
and
V. A. Rogozkin, D. Sc.
Director of Leningrad Research Institute
for Physical Education
Leningrad, USSR

Series Editors:

Richard C. Nelson, Ph. D.
and
Chauncey A. Morehouse, Ph. D.
The Pennsylvania State University

University Park Press
Baltimore

UNIVERSITY PARK PRESS
International Publishers in Science and Medicine
233 East Redwood Street
Baltimore, Maryland 21202

Copyright © 1978 by University Park Press

Typeset by Everybodys Press
Manufactured in the United States of America by
The Maple Press Company.

Library of Congress Cataloging in Publication Data
Main entry under title:
Nutrition, physical fitness, and health.
(International series on sport sciences; v. 7) Includes index.
1. Physical fitness—Nutritional aspects. 2. Athletes—Nutrition. 3. Health.
I. Pařízková, Jana. II. Rogozkin, V. A. III. Series. [DNLM: 1. Nutrition.
2. Physical fitness. 3. Sport medicine. QT255.3 N976] RC1235.N87 613.2
78-5912
ISBN 0-8391-1263-7

Contents

Contributors

I.I. Alexandrov Leningrad Research Institute of Physical Education, prospect Dinamo 2., 197047 Leningrad, USSR

M. Apfelbaum Laboratoire de Physiologie, Hôpital Bichat, 170 Bld Ney, 75877 Paris, Cedex 18, France

J.D. Brooke Department of Human Kinetics, University of Guelph, College of Biological Science, Guelph, Ontario, Canada N1G 2W1

I. Celejowa Laboratory of Athlete Nutrition, Department of Hygiene Academy of Physical Education, 01-813 Warsaw, Poland

B. Chatterjee IDL Chemicals Limited, Research, Jamai-Osmania, Hyderabad - 500007, India

D.L. Costill Human Performance Laboratory, Ball State University, Muncie, Indiana 47306 USA

F. Duret Laboratoire de Physiologie, Hôpital Bichat, 170 Bld Ney, 75877 Paris, Cedex 18, France

J.V.G.A. Durnin Institute of Physiology, University of Glasgow, Glasgow W.2., Scotland

Z. Fejfar Cardiovascular Research Center, Institute of Clinical and Experimental Medicine, Budějovická 800, Prague 4-Krč, Czechoslovakia

A. Ferro-Luzzi Istituto Nazionale della Nutrizione, Via Lancisi 29, Roma 00116, Italy

H.L. Garrett Department of Physical Education, University of Kentucky, Lexington, Kentucky USA

E. Hultman Department of Clinical Chemistry, Karolinska Institutet, Serafimerlasarettet, Hantverkargatan 2, S-112 21 Stockholm, Sweden

K.A. Laritcheva Institute of Nutrition, Academy of Medical Sciences, Ustinskyi proezd 2/14, Moscow ZH-240, USSR

G.V. Mann Department of Biochemistry, School of Medicine, Vanderbilt University, Nashville, Tennessee 37232 USA

R. Masironi Cardiovascular Diseases Unit, World Health Organization, Avenue Appia, 1211 Geneva, Switzerland

D.S. Miller Queen Elisabeth College, London W8 7AH, England

A. Nadamuni Naidu National Institute of Nutrition, Indian Council of Medical Research, Jamai-Osmania, Hyderabad- 500007, India

L. Namyslowshi Institute of Biomedical Sciences, Academy of Physical Education, 01-813 Warsaw, Poland

B.S. Narasinga Rao National Institute of Nutrition & Indian Council of Medical Research, Jamai-Osmania, Hyderabad- 500007, India

N.G. Norgan Department of Human Sciences, University of Technology, Loughborough, Leicestershire LE 11 3TU, England

F. Ohta Division of Health Promotion, National Institute of Nutrition, Toyamacho 1, Shinjiku-ku, Tokyo, Japan

K. Ošancová Center of Food Hygiene and Nutrition, Institute of Hygiene and Epidemiology, Šrobárova 48, Prague 10-Vinohrady, Czechoslovakia

S. Oshima Division of Health Promotion, National Institute of Nutrition, Toyamacho 1, Shinjiku-ku, Tokyo, Japan

J. Pařízková Research Institute, Faculty of Physical Education, Charles University, Újezd 450, 11807 Prague 1., Czechoslovakia

A. Reinberg Laboratoire de Chronobiologie, Fondation Rotschild, 29 rue Manin, 75019 Paris, France

V.A. Rogozkin Leningrad Research Institute for Physical Education, prospect Dinamo 2., 197047 Leningrad, USSR

B. Saltin August Krogh Institute, University of Copenhagen, 13 Universitetsparken, 2100 Copenhagen Ø, Denmark

K. Satyanarayana National Institute of Nutrition, Indian Council of Medical Research, Jamai-Osmania, Hyderabad - 500007, India

N.N. Shishina Leningrad Research Institute for Physical Education, prospect Dinamo 2., 197047 Leningrad, USSR

V.I. Shubin Institute of Nutrition, Academy of Medical Sciences of USSR, Ustinskyi proezd 2/14, Moscow ZH-240, USSR

P.V. Smirnov Institute of Nutrition, Academy of Medical Sciences of USSR, Ustinskyi proezd 2/14, Moscow ZH-240, USSR

J. Šonka Laboratory for Endocrinology and Metabolism, Faculty of Medicine, Charles University, U nemocnice 1., Prague 2-12821 Czechoslovakia

S. Suzuki Division of Health Promotion, National Institute of Nutrition, Toyamacho 1, Shinjiku-ku, Tokyo, Japan

E. Tsuji Division of Health Promotion, National Institute of Nutrition, Toyamacho 1, Shinjiku-ku, Tokyo, Japan

K. Tsuji Division of Health Promotion, National Institute of Nutrition, Toyamacho 1, Shinjiku-ku, Tokyo, Japan

A. Venerando Istituto di Medicina della Sport, Via dei Campi Sportivi 46, 00197 Roma, Italy

W. Wirths Lehrstuhl für Angewandte Ernährungsphysiologie, Römerstr. 164, 5300 Bonn 1, Federal Republic of Germany

J. Wykurz Department of Nutrition and Hygiene, Institute of Social Medicine, Medical Academy, Warsaw, Poland

N.I. Yalovaya National Institute of Nutrition, Academy of Medical Sciences of USSR, Ustinskyi proezd 2/14, Moscow ZH-24, USSR

Preface

Interrelationships between nutrition and physical activity, representing the most important aspects of energy input and output, have become a topic of increasing interest because of their mutual dependence and the important role of both in terms of their optimal or impaired balance in the functional capacity, fitness, and health status of the organism. In 1975, at the occasion of the Xth International Congress of Nutrition in Kyoto, Japan, a special committee devoted to these subjects was established by the International Union of Nutritional Sciences (IUNS), which is associated with UNESCO. The aim of this Committee is to collect all available information on research in this particular area, to encourage or organize scientific meetings, and to summarize and define recommendations for practice. The present volume is a result of this Committee's activities.

Research work in nutrition, functional capacity, and fitness has been developing successfully in the past years, as witnessed by numerous international meetings—e.g., regular conferences on "Nutrition, Dietetics and Sport" in Bordighera in 1976 and Rome in 1973, the "International Symposium on Athletes Nutrition" in Leningrad in 1975, the special symposium on "Nutrition and Physical Fitness in Man" held within the framework of the Xth International Congress of Nutrition, and many others. There already exist many surveys and monographs that deal with this problem, but new information is accumulating and further research is underway. Therefore, this volume was compiled.

Relationships between caloric intake and output, nutrition, and physical activity have had an important impact on growth and development from the very beginning of life. A characteristic motor pattern and volume of physical activity is claimed to be related to special body physique (obviously also to a special metabolic pattern and functional capacity) in infants, as well as in children and adolescents. This applies also to adult age groups, and has great importance not only for general fitness but also for performance capacity from the professional point of view, with special relevance for the economic production and health prognosis in later periods of life. These problems have been studied in various surveys of human subjects and analyzed in greater detail in fundamental research in experimental models with laboratory animals.

Diet that is quantitatively and qualitatively deficient, and overnutrition, i.e., too abundant and inadequately balanced diet, are serious problems of malnutrition, especially when they are not maintained in a proper relation to the level of physical activity and muscular work. Obviously, protein energy malnutrition and its consequences for somatic and mental development, as well as functional capacity, is a most important problem in developing countries, but hyperalimentation accompanied by hypokinesia is considered to be one of the most important risk factors for cardiovascular disease in industrially developed countries, according to the World Health Organization (WHO). Unfortunately, along with technological advances, they are transferred to certain social strata in other areas of the world.

Therefore, we have tried to find evidence for the aspects mentioned, all of which are assumed to be very important tasks for the IUNS committee. Adequate criteria for optimal nutrition in special ecological situations have to be defined more accurately, including desirable functional capacity and health prognosis. Standard values of height and weight for individual age categories from developed countries are not the optimum for all places in the world, but they are often used as such. This area of research deserves increased emphasis.

Throughout the world, champion sport attracts more interest than any other social phenomenon. Nutrition of athletes related to special kinds or phases of training and competition for different age categories is a topic given enormous attention by sport medical doctors, coaches, and trainers. Since ancient times, there have existed recommendations and recipes for athletes that were assumed to ensure the optimal level of performance; however, conclusive decisions have never been reached, and it remains a task for many laboratories and institutes around the world.

An attempt was made in this publication to indicate some of the more general aspects that make the interrelationships between nutrition, physical activity, and fitness so important. The role of individual nutrients, water, and electrolytes is discussed and documented by experimental data gained both in human subjects and laboratory models with animals. This volume, which was arranged in a brief period of time, does not aspire to cover the entire area. It rather provides some information about more recent progress in the research in nutrition and exercise, which is surely not complete and is sometimes contradicting. However, this is characteristic of the situation at present; discrepancies are often attributable to the fact that exercise is taken generally, i.e., the pecularities of dynamic or static work loads are not considered.

Many renowned research workers were asked to contribute; not all were able or willing to fulfill our request, and those who did prepared their contribution in a way corresponding to their ideas, which was fully respected. The intention was not to interfere with the area of exercise biochemistry, although some overlapping was unavoidable. This research area is excellently covered by a group of distinguished scientists who presented their data at the occasion of the International Symposia of Exercise Biochemistry (Brussels, 1968; Magglingen, 1973; Quebec 1976) and elsewhere. Some of these research workers who are interested more in the impact of special diets nevertheless contributed to this volume.

Let us hope this collection of papers will not only give summarized information, but will also constitute another step in the development of studies concerning nutrition, physical activity, and performance, and will encourage future research in this field so important in practical life.

J. Pařízková
V. A. Rogozkin

NUTRITION, PHYSICAL FITNESS, AND HEALTH

Metabolic Aspects of Performance Capacity

Food Intake and Energy Utilization

D. S. Miller

This chapter is limited to data on man, because man exhibits important differences from other species. It is not implied that man can cheat the general principles of physiology, biochemistry, or even the laws of thermodynamics—man simply exhibits far wider genetic and behavioral variations than do the animal species normally studied by science. There are many reasons for this. Whereas laboratory, farm, and domestic animals have been selected for specific characteristics, there are strong taboos in all human cultures that prevent such selection from taking place in man. Farm livestock have been developed with a high efficiency of energy utilization for the economic benefit of the farmer, and the laboratory rat is so genetically uniform as to be often homozygous. It could be argued that natural selection in man might have favored those individuals who were good utilizers of food such that they were more resistant to famine, but such individuals would have become obese in times of plenty, and thus less able to avoid the hazards of primordial predators. It is not surprising, therefore, that we find among any human population a wide range of energy utilization not found among domesticated animals. Further unique features of man's existence are an extended period of development and longevity. Domesticated animals reach maturity within a year or two, and few studies on middle-aged or old laboratory animals are recorded. On the other hand, man takes 20 years to reach maturity, and can maintain his mature weight within narrow limits for an additional 50 years. The most interesting aspect of this ability is that he can do this on a wide range of food intakes, and it is this factor that makes the statement of human energy requirements so difficult.

There is much controversy today as to the nature of homeostatic controls for the regulation of energy balance in man. Undoubtedly controls of food intake exist in man as in other animals, but it would seem that these are coarse controls, easily overridden by the higher centers of the brain. One has only to compare the laboratory rat eating his cubed diet for months on end with the gourmet entertaining his friends and colleagues at lunch, working through an extensive menu of delectable dishes, to realize that human food has sensual, social, cultural, and economic values quite apart from its nutritional content. This has resulted in the growing belief that control of the efficiency of utilization of energy must also be important in man if we are to explain the ability of some of us to maintain weight over long periods of time without even trying.

VARIATIONS IN FOOD INTAKE

The central problem in this field is to explain how apparently similar individuals can maintain energy balance on widely differing food intakes. Widdowson (1962) has demonstrated that for any 20 people of the same age, sex, and occupation, one individual could be found who was eating twice as much as another person. She also stated that there are some infants who eat even more than some adults. Since these results were originally published, all dietary surveys on individuals have shown a similar variation irrespective of the length of the study or the level of the energy intake. How is this possible? Widdowson's data indicate that the explanation is not to be found in variations in body weight (despite the recent recommendations of FAO/WHO, 1974), because expressing the figures in terms of intake per kg body weight shows an equally wide variation. In studies of different populations—whether from different countries or from different social classes within those countries, it is shown that the mean energy intakes of groups of adults also show wide variation. For example, the mean intake of male Americans is more than 3,000 kcal, but that of Ethiopians is only 2,000 kcal per day. It is difficult to believe that the explanation of these differences is attributable to differences in physical activity, because Americans live in an affluent, labor-saving society, and Ethiopians are subsistence farmers. However, it is clear that the explanation must lie in differences in energy expenditure, and that this results largely from differences in heat production—i.e., thermogenesis. Increased thermogenesis can arise from a number of causes (Miller, 1975): it may be induced by cold, stress, drugs in common use, and also by diet. Dietary-induced thermogenesis is the manifestation of poor food utilization; it has been variously described as Specific Dynamic Action, the thermic effect of food, and luxuskonsumption, but these terms have led to much confusion in the literature, and until the phenomenon is properly understood, the general term, dietary-induced thermogenesis (DIT), should be used.

Experimental Overfeeding

There is now a mass of evidence to show that weight changes in response to overeating in man are not always positive and cannot be predicted by simply dividing the excess energy intake by a factor representing the energy density of adipose tissue. The earliest experiments were by Neumann (1902) and by Gulick (1922). Both conducted experiments on themselves continuously for several years and demonstrated that their body weights could be maintained on energy intakes 40% above their customary intake. In the author's own experiments (Miller and Mumford, 1967), 49 subjects have now been overfed. They have been given a variety of diets for periods up to 8 weeks. The customary food intake of each subject was measured during the week previous to overfeeding. During the experimental weeks they were encouraged to eat as much food as possible, but in any case a minimum of 1,000 kcal extra each day. Initially, the effects of eating diets of high and low protein contents were compared, but subsequent experiments involving comparisons of nibbling (14 meals/day) and gorging (2 meals/day), high and low sodium diets, and diets containing a high proportion of sucrose or starch were undertaken. With the exception of those subjects fed two meals a day, there was a marked adaptation to the increased energy intake such that the rate of gain decreased throughout the experiment. This resulted in very small weight gains compared with the extra food consumed, and most of this weight was put on during the first week of overfeeding. Some individuals consumed 10,000 excess kcal/week and showed a weight loss.

These experiments have been repeated by a number of workers, but the most notable are the marathon overfeeding experiments of Simms and co-workers (1973). They persuaded their subjects to consume 7–10,000 kcal/day for periods of 200 days or more—an excess of food intake of approximately 1 gigacalorie (million kcal). The subjects were expected to increase their body weights by 20–25%, and measurements were made of the energy cost of maintenance before and after overeating. However, not all subjects were equally successful in gaining weight. Some reached their goal with difficulty, but others failed to gain even though they were consuming more than those who gained readily. Their data for the energy cost of maintenance was for the overfed 2,700 kcal/m^2, compared with 1,800 kcal/m^2 before the experiment.

There are a number of possibilities to account for the lack of weight gain in all these experiments. Reduced digestibility of food and increased physical activity are easily eliminated by making the appropriate measurements. However, there has been some controversy as to the relative importance of changes in body composition and increased heat production. It now seems apparent that some changes in body composition occur initially, and that a period of a week or two is required for adaptation. Subsequently, heat production is increased. This has been established both by measuring oxygen consumption and by direct calorimetry.

Experimental Underfeeding

Since the authoritative work of Keys and his co-workers (1950), it has been established that energy expenditure decreases during starvation. Quite apart from a reduction in physical activity, both the basal metabolic rate and dietary-induced thermogenesis are depressed. However, only recently have these variables been measured on individuals who ordinarily maintain weight on low energy intakes as distinct from starved volunteers. Of particular interest are those obese individuals who claim to be able to lose weight on recommended diets that barely equal their calculated requirements for basal metabolic rate. Miller and Parsonage (1975) have just completed such a study. The subjects were selected from slimming clubs and were incarcerated in an isolated country house and fed 1,500 kcal /day. Their luggage was searched and their car keys removed. A full program was arranged, and they were observed throughout the 3 weeks of the trial. Although 19 of the subjects did lose weight, nine maintained weight within ± 1 kg, and two actually gained weight. There was a good correlation between weight change and basal metabolic rate, and the group as a whole was 18% below Harris-Benedict standards (range +8% to −47%). Similar correlations were found between daily energy expenditures and changes in weight. However, it is not clear whether such individuals are prone to obesity because of their low metabolic rates or whether their low metabolic rates are a result of their consuming low energy intakes. Nevertheless, it does establish that within a normal human population there are individuals maintaining weight on extremely low intakes, and they can do this by a severe reduction in energy expenditure.

Dietary-Induced Thermogenesis

From the previously described experiment, it is apparent that the wide range of observed food intakes in any population may be explained by a similar wide range of energy expenditure, even when the level of physical activity is held constant. There is no doubt that this range partly results from differences in basal metabolic rate that can be reduced on low intakes and may be elevated in overfeeding. Another important factor is the magnitude of dietary-induced thermogenesis. In many experiments this is manifested simply by differences in the energy cost of simple activities such as standing, sitting, and walking, which occupy most of our day. However, carefully controlled experiments show that not only is resting energy expenditure elevated after feeding and in proportion to the size of the meal, but that the effect is potentiated by exercise (Miller, Mumford, and Stock, 1967) and influenced by the nutritional status as indicated by previous diet (Miller and Wise, 1975). A recent study of six obese and six anorexic patients is relevant (Miller, Green, and Wynn, 1975). Both groups had been put on remedial diets for some time before measurements of dietary-induced thermogenesis were made. The underfed obese increased their metabolic rate in response to a standard meal by only 11%, whereas the overfed anorectics increased by 25%.

In summary, habitual large eaters may show elevated basal metabolic rates, high dietary-induced thermogenesis, and high minute energy costs for everyday activities. Conversely, these variables are low in habitual small eaters.

ENERGY REQUIREMENTS

It is popular for governments and international agencies to prescribe recommended dietary allowances for most nutrients. These may be based on normal intakes of a healthy population or on experimentally determined physiological minima plus some safety factor. In the case of energy, there is a very real dilemma because of the wide range of energy utilization, and all committees so far have only stated average requirements for groups of individuals. Unfortunately, this can only be of limited value, because it is impossible to ascertain whether food is distributed according to the physiological requirements of individuals. For example, it is often important to estimate the number of undernourished individuals in a population to ascertain the seriousness of a problem, and there is no standard for this calculation on the basis of food consumption. This is no ivory-tower exercise, because undernutrition is almost certainly the most serious nutritional problem in the world today, and it is important to quantify it on humanitarian grounds and for logistic reasons. It is also politically important.

From what is now known about adaptations to high and low caloric intakes, it would seem that there is a range over which energy expenditure may be adjusted to ensure energy balance. Below this range there will be an inevitable loss of body substance, and above it, fat will accumulate. The range for normal individuals is quite wide, but it may depend upon genetic factors. Future committees might be more useful if they were to estimate the range. For instance, they might decide that it was injurious to health for a man to consume less than

1,500 kcal /day *or* more than 3,000 kcal /day. Such a recommendation would have far-reaching effects, because it would remove much of the world food problem and direct aid to the really needy. Later committees might feel that 3,000 kcal /day is too high a maximum, because there is a low prevalence of diseases of civilization—e.g., obesity—among populations where few individuals consume more than 2,500 kcal /day. Adaptations to low intakes are known to increase longevity; adaptations to high intakes may carry a penalty.

REFERENCES

FAO/WHO. 1974. Energy and Protein Requirements. WHO Technical Report Series, no. 522, Geneva.

Gulick, A. 1922. A study of weight regulation in the adult human body during overnutrition. Am. J. Physiol. 60: 3.

Keys, A., Brosek, J., Henschel, A., Michelson, O., and Taylor, H. L. 1950. The Biology of Human Starvation. Minnesota Press, Minneapolis.

Miller, D. S. 1975. Thermogenesis in everyday life. In E. Jequier (ed.), Regulation of Energy Balance in Man. Editions Médecine et Hygiene, Geneva.

Miller, D. S., Green, E., and Wynn, V. 1975. Oxygen consumption of obese and anorectic patients. Proc. Nutr. Soc. 34: 14A.

Miller, D. S., and Mumford, P. M. 1967. Gluttony, I. An experimental study of overfeeding low and high protein diets. Am. J. Clin. Nutr. 20: 1212.

Miller, D. S., Mumford, P. M. and Stock, M. J. 1967. Gluttony. II. Thermogenesis in overeating man. Am. J. Clin. Nutr. 20: 1223.

Miller, D. S., and Parsonage, S. 1975. Resistance to slimming. Lancet i: 773.

Miller, D. S., and Wise, A. 1975. Exercise and dietary induced thermogenesis. Lancet i: 1290.

Neumann, R. A. 1902. Experimentelle Beitrage zur Lehre von dem täglichen Nahrungsbedarfes Menschen unter besonderer Beruchsichtigung der notwendigen Eiweissmenge. Arch. Hyg. 45: 1.

Simms, E. A. H., Danforth, E., Horton, E. S., Bray, G. A., Glennon, J. A., and Saland, L. B. 1973. Endocrine and metabolic effects of experimental obesity in man. Rec. Prog. Horm. Res. 29: 457.

Widdowson, E. M. 1962. Nutritional individuality. Proc. Nutr. Soc. 21: 121.

Liver as a Glucose Supplying Source During Rest and Exercise, with Special Reference to Diet

E. Hultman

The liver is generally recognized as the only significant source for blood glucose in the post-prandial state. It is also well known today that in situations with increased energy demand, such as exercise, the glucose output from the liver is increased. The increase is accomplished both by the pathways of glycogenolysis and gluconeogenesis. The importance of these mechanisms for work performance capacity was demonstrated by Issekutz, Issekutz, and Nach (1970), among others, who showed that dogs performing endurance exercise ceased to work as soon as the supply of newly released glucose from the liver became inadequate. Pronounced decreases in blood glucose concentrations have also been observed in man at the end of prolonged exercise periods, limiting the performance capacity (Bergström, Hultman, and Roch-Norlund, 1967).

THE SIZE OF THE LIVER GLYCOGEN STORE

The liver glycogen store in normal man in the post-prandial state after normal mixed diet was found to be 270 mmole glucose units per kg liver, with range values of 87–460 mmole (Figure 1) (Nilsson, 1973; Hultman and Nilsson, 1975). With a normal liver weight of 1.8 kg, this glycogen store would correspond to a mean of 490 mmole glucose units. The size of this glycogen store varies with the preceding diet from 900 mmole in the whole liver after a carbohydrate-rich diet to 67 mmole totally after starvation or a normocaloric intake of carbohydrate-poor diet (Table 1).

This work was supported by grants from the Swedish Medical Research Council, Project No. B76-19X-2647-08B.

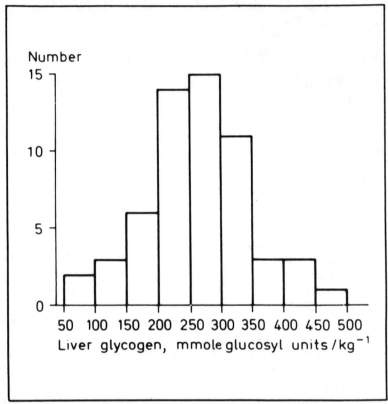

Figure 1. Liver glycogen content in the post-absorptive state in normal man, determined in tissue obtained by percutaneous liver biopsy.

LIVER GLUCOSE PRODUCTION AT REST

After a Normal Mixed Diet

The net release of glucose from the liver in normal man in the post-prandial state has been determined to be 0.8–1.1 mmole per min, or approximately 1 mole per day. This amount covers the energy needs of the brain and obligatory glycolytic tissues in the body (Cahill and Owen, 1968). The glucose is produced via two pathways: gluconeogenesis, in which lactate, pyruvate, glycerol, and amino acids are utilized for glucose production, and glycogenolysis.

From studies of uptake of the gluconeogenic precursors by the liver, it has been determined that the maximum production via gluconeogenesis in the normal resting state is approximately 25–30% of the glucose output (Wahren et al., 1971b; Nilsson, Fürst, and Hultman, 1973).

Table 1. Glycogen stores and glucose metabolism in the liver at rest in relation to preceding diet[a]

Stores and metabolism	After mixed diet	After CHO-poor diet, 1–10 days	After CHO-rich diet, 1–15 days
Glycogen content (mmole glucose units(kg liver)			
mean	270	37	467
range	87–460	12–73	267–624
Glucose release (mmole/min)			
mean	0.87[b]	0.30[b]	0.95
Glycogenolysis rate (mmole glucose/min)			
mean	0.52[c]	0	0.50[d]
Gluconeogenesis rate (mmole/min)			
mean	0.31[e]	0.30[e]	0.45[d]

[a] The diet period before determination of liver glucose metabolism was 3–4 days.

[b] From Nilsson, Furst, and Hultman (1973).

[c] Determined by repeated glycogen determination in liver biopsy samples (Nilsson and Hultman, 1973).

[d] Glycogenolysis rate calculated as difference between glucose release and gluconeogenesis rate, which was determined as uptake of lactate, pyruvate, glycerol, and alanine by the splanchnic area.

[e] Determined as gluconeogenesis using urea output by the liver as a measure of amino acid utilization (Nilsson, Furst, and Hultman, 1973).

Direct determination of glycogen content in the liver in repeatedly sampled tissue showed a glycogenolysis rate of 0.30 mmole glucose units per kg liver per min, or 0.54 mmole per min in the whole liver (Figure 2). The measured rate of glycogen degradation in the liver would correspond to the remaining two-thirds of the total hepatic glucose release (Hultman and Nilsson, 1971; Nilsson and Hultman, 1973) (Table 1).

From the figure of glycogenolysis rate, it can be calculated that the mean glycogen store of the liver (490 mmole glucose units per 1.8 kg liver) should last for 15–16 hr, and should be completely empty after one day of starvation. This result was confirmed in four subjects in whom liver biopsies were taken after 24 and 38 hr of starvation (Hultman and Nilsson, 1973).

After Starvation or a Carbohydrate-Poor Diet

In subjects maintained on a carbohydrate-poor, normocaloric diet, the liver glycogen content showed the same low values as after 24 hr of

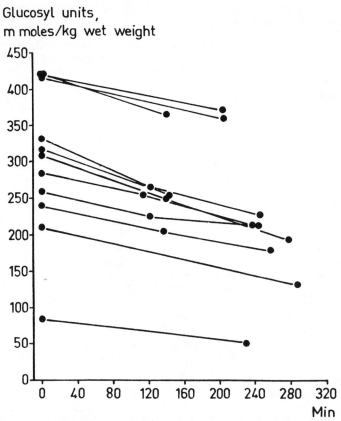

Figure 2. Liver glycogen content during short-term starvation. Tissue samples obtained in the morning in the post-absorptive state and after 2 and 4 hr further rest and starvation. The mean glycogen decreases corresponded to 0.30 mmole glucosyl units · kg⁻¹ · min⁻¹.

starvation. Continued diet regimen, with high protein and fat intake during 10 days, gave the same low glycogen content during the whole observation period (12−73 mmole glucose units per kg liver, or totally, 20−130 mmole per 1.8 kg) (Figure 3, Table 3.)

In liver vein catheterization studies, the uptake of gluconeogenic substrates and the glucose production was determined in the post-adsorptive state and after 3−6 days of carbohydrate-poor diet. The results are presented in Table 4, and show that the uptake of gluconeogenic substrates was unchanged. Because the liver glycogen content was close to zero after the carbohydrate-poor diet, glycogenolysis was unlikely to occur, and the expected result was thus a decrease in total glucose production from the liver. This was also confirmed by the direct measurement of glucose output from the splanch-

Table 2. Liver glycogen content during short-term starvation[a]

Glycogen, glucosyl units (mmole/kg wet liver tissue)	Subjects										
	BO	UT	GD	SS	TL	LT	BG	LR	GO	AÅ	KE
Basal	419	316	308	284	259	210	241	420	416	335	87
Approximately 2 hr further starvation	366	254	250	257	227		206			265	
Approximately 4 hr further starvation			196	212	213	133	179	374	362	229	51
Decrease per min	0.38	0.43	0.40	0.30	0.19	0.27	0.24	0.23	0.27	0.43	0.16

[a] Tissue samples obtained by repeated needle biopsy (Nilsson and Hultman, 1973). Basal mean was 300 (0.30 decrease per min, and basal SEM was 30.5 (0.029 decrease per min).

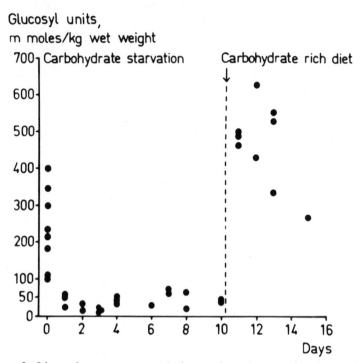

Figure 3. Liver glycogen content during prolonged starvation or supply of carbohydrate-poor (CHO-poor) diet followed by carbohydrate refeeding.

nic area in the catheterization study (Table 4). In spite of a 70% decrease in glucose production from the liver, only a small decrease in blood sugar was observed (Nilsson, Fürst, and Hultman, 1973). This infers that a corresponding reduction of glucose uptake by extrasplanchnic tissue must have occurred. The decreased glucose uptake corresponds to the change from glucose to ketone body utilization by the brain (Owen et al., 1967; Gottstein et al., 1971; Krebs et al., 1971; Williamson, Bates, and Krebs, 1971; Sugden and Newsholme, 1973; Flatt et al, 1974). A pronounced increase in β-hydroxy-butyrate and acetoacetate production by the liver was also found after the period of carbohydrate-poor diet (Nilsson, Fürst, and Hultman, 1973).

After Carbohydrate-Rich Diet

Carbohydrate-rich diet given after total or carbohydrate starvation resulted in an immediate increase in liver glycogen content after only one day of refeeding. The glycogen content was as high as 469–513 mmole per kg liver. Also, the hepatic glucose release was higher than after the carbohydrate-poor diet (see Table 1). Hepatic uptake of lactate and alanine was increased, and the blood concentrations of these substrates were higher than after carbohydrate-poor diet (Table 5).

Table 3. Effects of prolonged starvation or supply of carbohydrate-poor diet followed by carbohydrate refeeding . Liver glycogen content and blood glucose levels

		Glycogen (mmole glucosyl units/kg wet liver tissue)															
		Days of total starvation or CHO-poor diet										Days of CHO-rich diet				
Subjects	Basal	1	2	3	4	5	6	7	8	9	10	1	2	3	4	5
LA[a]	155	24	15	21								513				
TW[a]	345	48														
JS[b]	98				33			60			42	462		552		
KE[b]	298				44			73			39	496		526		
MA[b]	213			12					64				624			
CF[b]	401			15					17							
MF[b]	112						30						424			
EJ[b]	230	55	32		48									336	267	
Mean	232															
Blood glucose (mmole/liter) mean	5.10	4.58	3.92	3.92	3.86	3.78	4.68	4.00	4.50	4.17	4.25	5.01	4.91	4.61		4.59

[a] Total starvation.
[b] CHO-poor diet.

Table 4. Hepatic glucose production from glycogenolysis and from gluconeogenesis after different diets[a]

Production source	Normal diet (mmole/min)	CHO-poor diet (mmole/min)
Glycogen[b]	0.54	0.00
Protein, calculated from urea production	0.15	0.13
Lactate	0.12	0.13
Glycerol	0.04	0.04
Total calculated glucose production	0.85	0.30
Directly determined glucose production	0.87	0.30

[a] Uptake of substrates and production of glucose were determined by liver vein catheterization after diet periods of 3−4 days.

[b] Glycogenolysis value was taken from Nilsson and Hultman (1973).

Substrate Control of Hepatic Glucose Release

The role of the gluconeogenic substrate for hepatic glucose release was studied in healthy volunteers. They were pretreated for 3 days with the carbohydrate-poor diet in order to empty the liver glycogen store. In the morning of Day 4, the liver vein catheterization was performed and the glucose production and substrate uptake over the splanchnic area was measured. After the basal period, an amino acid solution with high alanine content was infused at a rate of 1.76 mmole amino acids per min (0.7−1.0 mmole as alanine).

During the amino acid infusion, the rate of glucose release increased to 0.55 mmole per min. This increase was paralleled by increased release of urea from the liver. Assuming the carbon skeleton in the deaminated amino acids was utilized as the substrate for

Table 5. Arterial concentrations of glucose and gluconeogenic substrates at rest, after CHO-poor diets, and after CHO-rich diets

Arterial concentration	CHO-poor	CHO-rich
(mmole/liter)	mean ± S.E.M.	mean ± S.E.M.
Glucose	4.29 ± 0.070	5.64 ± 0.063
Lactate	0.527 ± 0.013	0.861 ± 0.064
Pyruvate	0.036 ± 0.001	0.074 ± 0.009
Alanine	0.109 ± 0.012	0.327 ± 0.013
Glycerol	0.050 ± 0.010	0.042 ± 0.008

gluconeogenesis, the amino acids could account for 74% of the total glucose release during the period of amino acid infusion. Thus, increased availability of gluconeogenic substrates may increase glucose production by the liver.

LIVER GLYCOGEN SYNTHESIS

The effect of dietary carbohydrate on liver glycogen content is seen in Tables 1 and 3. The glycogen synthesis rates from different sugars have been studied by measuring the glycogen content before and after a standardized infusion of 5.6 mmole hexose per kg body weight per hr during 4 hr. The infusion was performed in the post-adsorptive state. The synthesis rate was 0.3 mmole glucose units per min per kg liver during the 4-hr period of glucose infusion (Nilsson and Hultman, 1974). The same synthesis rate was found when glucose was given orally. When fructose was infused, the synthesis rate increased by 300% to 1.1 mmole per kg liver per min (Figure 4).

The observed rate of glycogen formation during the hexose infusion is of the same order of magnitude as the maximum rate of glucose conversion to glycogen in rat liver in situ reported by Krebs and coworkers (1974), and to an estimated liver glycogen synthesis rate of 0.5 mmole glucose units per kg liver per min in intact rats during the feeding period (Potter and Ono, 1961).

As described earlier, the rapid fructose infusion gave rise to both a blood lactate increase (Bergström, Hultman, and Roch-Norlund, 1968) and a degradation of ATP in liver tissue (Mäenpää, Raivio, and Kekomäki, 1968; Kekomäki, Raivio, and Mäenpää, 1970; Woods, Eggleston, and Krebs, 1970; Bode et al., 1971, 1973; Hultman, Nilsson, and Sahlin, 1975).

Table 6. Glucose release from the liver after 3 days of CHO-poor diet with and without amino acid infusion (1.5 mmole/min)[a]

Hepatic glucose production source	Before infusion (mmole glucose/min)	During amino acid infusion (mmole glucose/min)
Amino acids (urea)	0.14	0.39
Lactate	0.13	0.10
Glycerol	0.04	0.04
Total calculated	0.31	0.53
Determined by liver vein catheterization	0.30	0.55

[a] Furst, Guarnieri, and Hultman (1971).

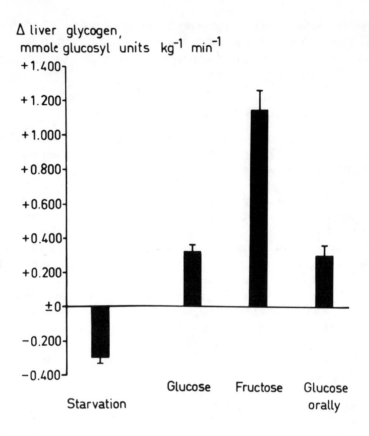

Figure 4. Liver glycogen degradation or synthesis rate during a 4-hr period with and without hexose infusion or peroral glucose administration. The amount hexose given was 5.6 mmole per kg body weight per hr.

HEPATIC GLUCOSE PRODUCTION
DURING EXERCISE AFTER NORMAL MIXED DIET

Increased hepatic output of glucose has been shown in both animal and human studies by [^{14}C] studies and by direct measurement with catheterization technique. It has also been shown that the glucose output increases with increasing work load and also with the work time during the exercise period (Rowell, Masoro, and Spencer, 1965; Bergström et al., 1967; Hultman, 1967; Issekutz, Issekutz, and Nach, 1970; Rowell, 1971; Wahren et al., 1971a,b; Hultman and Nilsson, 1973). The largest outputs of glucose from the liver are invariably found at the end of an exercise performed with a high work load.

Total Hepatic Glucose Release During Exercise

In an early study from the author's laboratory (Hultman, 1967), the hepatic production of glucose was measured during rest and exercise. The exercise was performed on a bicycle ergometer at a load of 75% of the subjects' Vo_2 max with repeated bouts of work of 20 min duration. It was found that the hepatic glucose output increased from 0.80 mmole per min at rest to 1.94 mmole during the first work period, and to a mean of 3.13 mmole per min during the last period. Of the total energy expenditure during exercise, hepatic glucose, if burned completely to CO_2 and water, could account for 14% during the whole exercise period and for 19% at the end.

Similar but slightly higher figures for hepatic glucose utilization were reported by Wahren et al. (1971b). They were able to calculate the fraction of carbohydrate utilized by the exercising legs that were derived from blood-borne glucose by utilizing a combination of direct determination of hepatic glucose output and uptake of glucose over exercising leg muscles. They found that 28−37% of the total substrates oxidized by the muscle at the end of exercise was derived from blood glucose.

At low work intensities the rate of glucose release from the liver is lower. In a study by Ahlborg et al. (1974), the hepatic glucose release at rest was 0.82 mmole per min. After 90, 180, and 240 min of exercise the amounts released were 1.85, 1.92, and 1.46 mmole per min, respectively. This glucose release, if oxidized by the working muscles, would correspond to 41, 36, and 30%, respectively, of the total oxygen uptake by the muscles. Thus, it seems indisputable today that during exercise, the hepatic output of glucose is important as an energy source for the working muscles.

Glycogenolysis During Exercise

Direct measurements of the liver glycogen store were made by the percutaneous liver biopsy technique. A liver biopsy was taken in the morning in the post-prandial state after 1hr of bicycle exercise, and the glycogen content in the tissue specimen was compared with liver tissue obtained from a similar group of subjects after 1hr of rest in the post-prandial state. The mean liver glycogen content was found to be 125 mmole glucose units lower per kg liver after exercise than after rest. This decrease would correspond to an output of glucose from the liver of 2.08 mmole per kg liver per min from glycogenolysis. The observed value fits surprisingly well with data of total output of hepatic glucose during exercise found by measurement in liver vein catheterization studies, i.e., 2.4−3.1 mmole per min (Hultman, 1967) and 2.2−3.8 mmole per min (Wahren et al., 1971b).

Gluconeogenesis During Exercise

Maximum gluconeogenesis during exercise was calculated from total uptake of gluconeogenic substrate (lactate, pyruvate, glycerol, and amino acids) by the splanchnic area. Thus, Wahren et al. (1971a, b) found a maximum gluconeogenic rate corresponding to 6−11% of the total hepatic glucose release at the end of a hard exercise. Of the gluconeogenic substrates taken up both at rest and during exercise, lactate is quantitatively the dominating one. At rest and during exercise at low to moderate work loads, about 50% of the gluconeogenesis was derived from lactate. At increasing work loads the dominance of lactate as gluconeogenic substrate increases (Wahren et al., 1971a, b).

The other individual substrates are of quantitatively minor importance. Several amino acids are taken up by the splanchnic area, but only alanine showed a constant release from the working muscle tissue at all levels of work intensity. The splanchnic uptake of alanine during exercise exceeded that of all other amino acids (Felig and Wahren, 1971). However, at high work loads, less than 1% of the splanchnic glucose production could be attributed to the uptake of alanine (Wahren et al., 1971b). At low work loads, during work periods of several hours duration, the uptake of alanine could correspond to a maximum of 4% of the total glucose production by the liver. The alanine shunt described by Felig and Wahren (1971) is therefore of quantitatively minor importance as a provider of energy substrate during exercise, especially at moderate to high work loads. On the other hand, both alanine and glutamine function as transporters of amino groups from working muscle to the splanchnic organs and to the kidneys.

DIETARY EFFECTS ON HEPATIC
GLUCOSE RELEASE DURING EXERCISE

In a study by Bergström, Hultman, and Roch-Norlund (1967), it was shown that the capacity to perform heavy exercise (75% of Vo_2 max) increased 300−400% when the preceding diet was changed from carbohydrate-poor to carbohydrate-rich. The diet regimen was kept for 3 days and was preceded by exhausting exercise designed to empty the muscle glycogen stores. It was found that the major effect of this exercise and diet regimen was to alter the muscle glycogen store at rest so that this store was lower than normal after the carbohydrate-poor diet, but was markedly elevated after the carbohydrate-rich diet. It was found that the performance capacity, measured as maximum work time at a constant work load, was correlated to the muscle glycogen store before the exercise. It was, however, observed that the blood glucose content was unchanged during exercise after the carbohydrate-rich diet, but decreased to subnormal values after the carbohydrate-poor diet. In two of the subjects, blood glucose values as low as 2 mmole per liter were observed at the end of exercise after the latter diet. The glucose level remained low for more than 1 hr after the end of exercise. Figure 5 shows the pronounced decrease in blood sugar after carbohydrate-poor diet and the lack of blood glucose increase after the end of the exercise. This lack of blood glucose increase after carbohydrate-poor diet was in contrast to the immediate elevation of blood glucose at the end of exercise after mixed diet or after the carbohydrate-rich diet. The subjects experienced headache and dizziness at the end of the exercise, probably caused by the hypoglycemia. Thus, these subjects seemed to have an inadequate hepatic glucose production, which apart from exhausted muscle glycogen stores, is likely to have contributed to limitation in work performance capacity after the period of carbohydrate-poor diet. Blood pyruvate and lactate levels were also lower during the exercise after the carbohydrate-poor diet compared to the levels after carbohydrate-rich diet.

This observation was followed up by a liver vein study (Hultman and Nilsson, 1973), in which two subjects exercised for 23 and 25 min, respectively, after pretreatment with carbohydrate-poor and carbohydrate-rich diets. Before and during the exercise period, splanch-

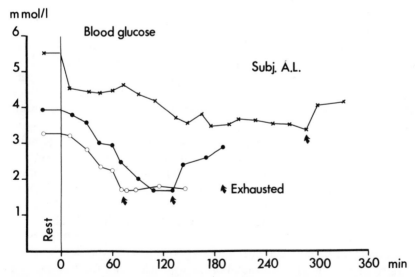

Figure 5. Blood glucose concentration before, during, and after exercise in one subject pretreated with different diets. × =carbohydrate-rich diet, ● =mixed diet, ○ =carbohydrate-poor diet, ← =denotes the point of exhaustion and end of exericise.

Table 7.   Splanchnic metabolism during rest and exercise in subjects pre-treated for 4 days with a CHO-rich and a CHO-poor diet[a]

Metabolite shift mean values	CHO-rich diet		CHO-poor diet	
(mmole/min)[b]	Rest	Work	Rest	Work
Glucose production	0.92	2.59	0.77	1.99
Lactate uptake	0.25	0.29	0.13	2.14
Pyruvate uptake	0.02	0.02	0.03	0.11
Glycerol uptake	0.04	0.04	0.11	0.13
α-amino acid uptake	0.61	0.07	0.80	0.50
Alanine uptake	0.13	0.04	0.18	0.14
Urea production	0.00	0.03	0.30	0.27
Oxygen uptake	2.43	2.70	2.44	4.46
Total glucose production (mmole)		57.55		49.50
Total uptake of metabolites (mmole)		9.00		72.20
Total calculated maximal gluconeogenesis (mmole)		4.50		36.10
Calculated glycogenolysis (mmole)		53.00 (8.6g)		13.40 (2.2g)

[a] Hultman and Nilsson (1973).

[b] Mean values calculated of three rest periods and four to six work periods for each subject. The total production of glucose and uptake of metabolites were calculated on the whole work period.

nic blood flow and metabolite shift were measured. The results, presented in Table 7, show an increased glucose release from the liver during exercise irrespective of the diet, but the preceding diet apparently had a pronounced effect on the pathways by which the liver glucose was produced. Thus, after the carbohydrate-rich diet, more than 90% of the glucose released during the exercise was derived via glycogenolysis. The corresponding value after the carbohydrate-poor diet was 25%. The remainder could be accounted for by gluconeogenesis from uptake of lactate, pyruvate, glycerol, and amino acids, for which substrates the extraction ratio over the splanchnic area was much higher after the carbohydrate-poor diet.

This study utilized sedentary subjects. They had high blood lactate concentrations during exercise, and consequently ample amounts of precursors for hepatic gluconeogenesis. To elucidate whether the same pattern of hepatic glucose metabolism was also valid for well-trained subjects, the study was repeated with five other subjects, all of whom exercised regularly. The subjects worked two times at the same relative work load (80% of V_{O_2} max) after 4 days on carbohydrate-poor and after 4 days on carbohydrate-rich diet. Liver and muscle metabolism were examined during the two work experiments. The results were similar in all the subjects. Data from two of the subjects are presented in Tables 8 and 9 and in Figures 6 and 7. The work schedule consisted of a work period of 20 min duration on a bicycle ergometer. This was followed by a 20-min "rest period" with continued pedaling at a low work load. Thereafter, the work was resumed at the predetermined work load and continued until exhaustion. The performance time was, as observed previously, longer after the carbohydrate-rich diet than after the carbohydrate-poor one. This could be attributable to two factors—an increased muscle glycogen store (see Table 8) and an expected increase in liver glycogen.

The liver glycogen stores after the two diets were not determined directly, but the hepatic glucose production as well as the uptake of gluconeogenic precursors were measured. From these figures it was possible to calculate the total amounts of liver glycogen utilized during exercise after carbohydrate-rich diet. These values were 322 and 197 mmole glucose units in the two subjects compared to 80 and 43, respectively, after carbohydrate-poor diet (Table 8). These figures should be compared to the liver glycogen stores observed after different diets, as shown in Table 1. The hepatic venous and arterial concentrations for glucose and gluconeogenic substrates after the two diets are shown in Figures 6 and 7. It can be seen that hepatic venous glucose concentration increases continuously after both the diets during the first work period and in the beginning of the second. At the end of the exercise a decrease is seen in hepatic venous glucose concentration, followed also by a decrease in arterial glucose content after the carbohydrate-poor diet. This was apparently caused by a decreased capacity by the liver to produce sufficient amounts of glucose after the diet with low carbohydrate content. The most pronounced metabolic effect of the dietary change was the alteration in pathways for liver glucose production. After the carbohydrate-rich diet, 96 and 91% of the hepatic glucose release was derived from glucogenolysis (Tables 8 and 9); after the carbohydrate-poor diet the corresponding values were 52 and 59%, respectively.

Of the gluconeogenic substrates utilized, lactate alone could account for 80% of the total de novo synthesis of glucose after the carbohydrate-poor diet. After the carbohydrate-rich diet, on the other hand, the uptake of lactate by the liver during exercise was extremely low (Figures 6 and 7), and pyruvate was actually released from the liver in this situation, while taken up at rest and during exercise after carbohydrate-poor diet (Table 9). Thus, it seems that when the liver

Table 8. Carbohydrate metabolism during exercise in two subjects, each working to exhaustion at same relative work load after 4 days with CHO-poor and CHO-rich diets

Factors	Subject TL		Subject SL	
	CHO-poor	CHO-rich	CHO-poor	CHO-rich
1. Total work time (min)	43.1	89.5	42.0	52.0
2. Work load (watts)	200	200	205	205
3. Rate of oxygen uptake (liters/min)	2.83	2.65	3.00	2.84
4. Calculated total CHO oxidized:[a]				
a. mmole glucose units	454.3	1,343.0	364.4	593.2
b. percent of oxygen uptake accounted for	50	80	37	58
5. Lactate accumulated at the end of exercise (mmole in total body water)[b]	94.5	81.3	85.2	177.0
6. Calculated total CHO utilized (mmole glucose units)[c]	501.55	1,383.9	407.0	681.7
7. Calculated total CHO output from hepatic glycogenolysis:[d]				
a. mmole glucose units	80.1	322.2	42.8	196.6
b. percent of total CHO utilized	16.0	23.3	10.5	28.8
8. Calculated total CHO output from muscle glycogenolysis:[e]				
a. mmole glucose units	421.5	1,061.7	364.2	485.1
b. percent of total CHO utilized	84.0	76.7	89.5	71.2
9. Glycogen content of quadriceps[f]				
a. before exercise (mmole glucose units/ kg muscle)	46.0	100.4	69.0	92.5
b. after exercise	6.8	10.1	14.8	20.4
10. Calculated amount of muscle depleted of glycogen by end of exercise (kg)[g]	10.8	11.7	6.7	6.7

[a] Calculated from O_2 uptake and RQ (in expired air).

[b] Arterial concentration of lactate at the end of exercise multiplied by 60% of body weight.

[c] Sum of 4a and 5.

[d] Total hepatic glucose release minus uptake of gluconeogenic substrates.

[e] Calculated as 6 minus 7. The calculation infers that the only important sources for carbohydrate utilization during exercise are the glycogen stores in liver and muscle. Gluconeogenic substrates such as lactate, pruvate, and part of alanine circulate between muscle and liver. Additional substrates contributing to the carbohydrate moiety are glycerol from triglycerides and some amino acids from muscle protein. The contribution of these substrates is of quantitatively minor importance.

[f] Determined in biopsy specimens, from the m. quadriceps femoris.

[g] 8/(9a-9b).

Table 9. Splanchnic carbohydrate metabolism during exercise after different diets

Metabolite shift mean values (mmole glucose equivalents/min)	CHO-poor diet		CHO-rich diet	
	Subject TL	Subject SL	Subject TL	Subject SL
Glucose production	3.57	1.74	3.76	4.17
Lactate uptake	1.33	0.57	0.14	0.33
Pyruvate uptake or release	0.15	0.02	−0.03	−0.03
Glycerol uptake	0.13	0.08	0.05	0.03
Alanine uptake	0.09	0.05	0.03	0.03
Calculated maximum gluconeogenesis rate	1.71	0.73	0.19	0.36
Calculated glycogenolysis rate	1.86	1.02	3.6	3.78
Glycogenolysis in % of hepatic glucose release	52.1	58.6	95.7	90.6

glycogen stores are large, almost all glucose needed during exercise is produced by glycogenolysis, and gluconeogenic precursors are poorly utilized at high work loads. If the liver glycogen store is small, the utilization of gluconeogenic precursors increases, and lactate is the quantitatively most important for glucose production.

Glucose production via gluconeogenesis needs energy, which in Table 7 can be seen as an increased oxygen uptake by the liver, and in Table 8 as an increased rate of total oxygen uptake. The rate of glucose production from gluconeogenesis is in some situations not sufficient to keep the blood glucose level normal, because pronounced hypo-glycemia has been observed at the end of exercise after carbohydrate-poor diets (Bergström et al., 1967).

SUMMARY

In summary, the liver glycogen store can be kept normal or high only when the diet is rich in carbohydrate. A normocaloric diet with low carbohydrate content will result in low liver glycogen stores within 1 or 2 days.

Liver glycogen is utilized during hard exercise—especially during prolonged periods of work, when the muscle glycogen store is decreasing. A high liver glycogen store will suffice for glucose production during prolonged severe exercise, and in this situation almost all the

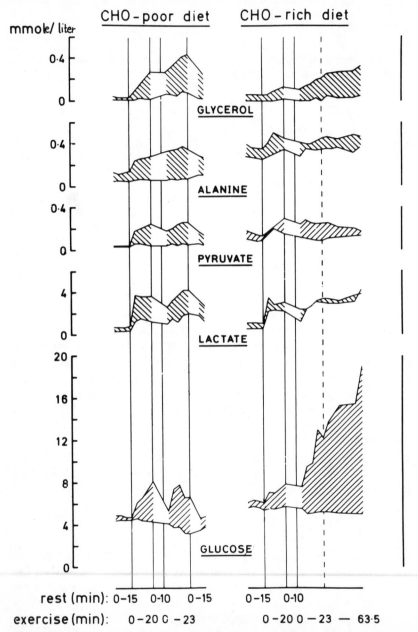

Figure 6. Arterial and hepatic venous contents of glucose and gluconeogenics substrates in Subject TL working with the same work load (200 watts) after carbohydrate-poor and carbohydrate-rich diets. \\\\ = hepatic extraction, //// = hepatic release.

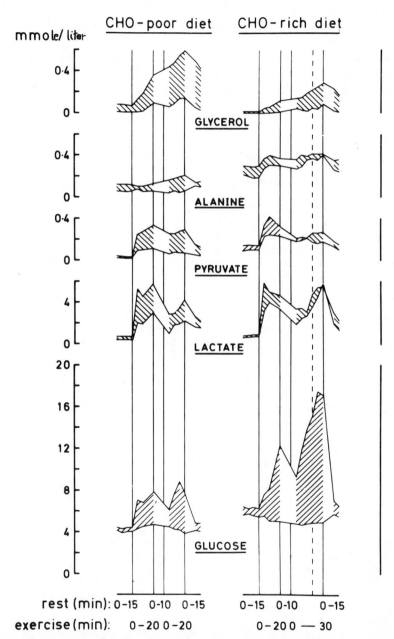

Figure 7. Arterial and hepatic venous contents of glucose and gluconeogenic substrates in Subject SL working with the same work load (205 watts) after carbohydrate-poor and carbohydrate-rich diets. \ \ \ \ = hepatic extraction, / / / / = hepatic release.

hepatic glucose release is derived from glycogenolysis. When the glycogen store is small, gluconeogenesis from lactate can partly replace the liver glycogen store as a source for blood glucose. The rate of gluconeogenesis can, however, be too low, resulting in hypoglycemia, which can limit the performance capacity when the carbohydrate intake has been insufficient to fill the liver glycogen store.

REFERENCES

Ahlborg, G., Felig, P., Hagenfeldt., L., Hendler, R., and Wahren, J. 1974. Substrate turnover during prolonged exercise in man. Splanchnic and leg metabolism of glucose, free fatty acids and amino acids. J. Clin. Invest. 53: 1080.

Bergström, K., Hermansen, L., Hultman, E., and Saltin, B. 1967. Diet, muscle glycogen and physical performance. Acta Physiol. Scand. 71: 140.

Bergström, J., Hultman, E., and Roch-Norlund, A. E. 1968. Lactic acid accumulation in connection with fructose infusion. Acta Med. Scand. 184: 359.

Bode, C., Schumacher, H., Goebell, H., Zelder, O., and Pelzer, H. 1971. Fructose induced depletion of liver adenine nucleotides in man. Horm. Metab. Res. 3: 289.

Bode, C., Zelder, O., Rumpelt, H. J., and Wittkamp, U. 1973. Depletion of liver adenosine phosphates and metabolic effects of intravenous infusion of fructose or sorbitol in man and in the rat. Europ. J. Clin. Invest. 3: 436.

Cahill, G. F., and Owen, O. E. 1968. In: F. Dickens, P. J., Randle, and Whelan (eds.), Carbohydrate Metabolism and Its Disorders, p. 497. Vol. 1. Academic Press, New York.

Felig, P., and Wahren, J. 1971. Amino acid metabolism in exercising man. J. Clin. Invest. 50: 2703.

Flatt, J. P., Blackburn, G. L., Randers, G., and Stanbury, J. B. 1974. Effects of ketone body infusion in hypoglycemic reaction in postabsorptive dogs. Metabolism 23: 151.

Fürst, P., Guarnieri, G., and Hultman, E. 1971. The effect of the administration of L-tryptophan on synthesis of urea and gluconeogenesis in man. Scand. J. Clin. Lab. Invest. 27: 183.

Gottstein, U., Müller, W., Berghoff, W., et al. 1971. Zur Utilisation von nichtverersten Fettsäuren und Ketonkörpern im Gehirn des Menschen. (For utilization of non-mineralized fatty acids and mixed ketones in human brains.) Klin. Wschr. 49: 406.

Hultman, E. 1967. Studies on muscle metabolism of glycogen and active phosphate in man with special reference to exercise and diet. Scand. J. Clin. Lab. Invest. 19 (suppl. 94).

Hultman, E., and Nilsson, L. H: son. 1971. Liver glycogen in man, effect of different diets and muscular exercise. In B. Pernow and B. Saltin, (eds.), Advances in Experimental Medicine and Biology, Vol. 11, pp. 143–151. Plenum Press, New York.

Hultman, E., and Nilsson, L. 1973. Liver glycogen as a glucose-supplying source during exercise. In J. Keul (ed.), Limiting Factors of Physical Performance. Int. Symp. at Gravenbuch, p. 179. Georg Thiemes Publishers, Stuttgart.

Hultman, E., and Nilsson, L. H:son. 1975. Factors influencing carbohydrate metabolism in man. Nutr. Metabol. 18 (suppl. 1): 45.

Hultman, E., Nilsson, L. H:son., and Sahlin, K. 1975. Adenine nucleotide content of human liver. Normal values and fructose-induced depletion. Scand. J. Clin. Lab. Invest. 35: 245.

Issekutz, B., Issekutz, A. C., and Nach, D. 1970. Mobilization of energy sources in exercising dogs. J. Appl. Physiol. 29: 691.

Kekomäki, M., Raivio, K. O., and Mäenpää, P. H. 1970. Interference with liver metabolism by D-fructose. Acta Anaesth. Scand. Suppl. 27: 114.

Krebs, H. A., Cornell, N. W., Lund, P., and Hems, L. R. 1974. Some aspects of hepatic energy metabolism. In F. Lundquist and N. Tygstrup (eds.), Regulation of Hepatic Metabolism, p. 549. Munksgaard, Copenhagen.

Krebs, H. A., Williamson, D. H., Bates, M. W., Page, M. A., and Hawkins, R. A. 1971. The role of ketone bodies in caloric homeostasis. Adv. Enzyme Regul. 9: 387.

Mäenpää, P. H., Raivio, K. O., and Kekomäki, M. P. 1968. Liver adenine nucleotides: Fructose-induced depletion and its effect on protein synthesis. Science 161: 1253.

Marliss, E. B., Acki, T. T., Pozefsky, T., Most, A. S., and Cahill, C. F. Jr. 1971. Muscle and splanchnic glutamine and glutamate metabolism in postabsorptive and starved man. J. Clin. Invest. 50: 814.

Nilsson, L. H:son. 1973. Liver glycogen content in man in the postabsorptive state. Scand. J. Clin. Lab. Invest. 32: 317.

Nilsson, L. H:son, Fürst, P., and Hultman, E. 1973. Carbohydrate metabolism of the liver in normal man under varying conditions. Scand. J. Clin. Lab. Invest. 32: 331.

Nilsson, L. H:son, and Hultman, E. 1973. Liver glycogen in man—The effect of total starvation or a carbohydrate-poor diet followed by carbohydrate refeeding. Scand. J. Clin. Lab. Invest. 32: 325.

Nilsson, L. H:son, and Hultman, E. 1974. Liver and muscle glycogen in man after glucose and fructose infusion. Scand. J. Clin. Lab. Invest. 33: 5.

Owen, O. E., Morgan, A. P., Kemp, H. G., Sullivan, J. M., Herrera, M. G., and Cahill, G. F. 1967. Brain metabolism during fasting. J. Clin. Invest. 46: 1589.

Potter, V. R., and Ono, T. 1961. Enzyme patterns in rat liver and Morris Hepatoma 5123 during metabolic transitions. Cold Spring Harbor Symp. Quant. Biol. 26: 355.

Ross, B. D., Hems, R., Freedland, R. A., and Krebs, H. A. 1967. Carbohydrate metabolism of the perfused rat liver. Biochem. J. 105: 869.

Rowell, L. B. 1971. The liver as an energy source in man during exercise. In B. Pernow and B. Saltin (eds.), Advances in Experimental Medicine and Biology, Vol. 11, p. 127. Plenum, New York.

Rowell, L. B., Masoro, E. J., and Spencer, M. J. 1965. Splanchnic metabolism in exercising man. J. Appl. Physiol, 20: 1032.

Sugden, P. O., and Newsholme, E. A. 1973. Activities of hexokinase, phosphofructokinase, 3-oxo acid coenzyme A-transferase and acetoacetylcoenzyme. A thiolase in nervous tissue from vertebrates and invertebrates. Biochem. J. 134: 97.

Wahren, J., Ahlborg, G., Felig, P., and Jorfeldt, L. 1971a. Glucose metabolism during exercise in man. In B. Pernow and B. Saltin (eds.), Advances in Experimental Medicine and Biology, Vol. II, p. 189. Plenum, New York.

Wahren, J., Felig, P., Ahlborg, G., and Jorfeldt, L. 1971b. Glucose metabolism during leg exercise in man. J. Clin. Invest. 50: 2715.

Williamson, D. H., Bates, M. W., and Krebs, H. A. 1971. Activities of enzymes involved in acetoacetate utilization in adult mammalian tissues. Biochem. J. 121: 41.

Woods, H. F., Eggleston, L. V., and Krebs, H. A. 1970. The cause of hepatic accumulation of fructose l-phosphate on fructose loading. Biochem. J. 119: 501.

Lactate Tolerance, Diet, and Physical Fitness

G. V. Mann, H. L. Garrett

It has been known since the work of A. V. Hill that lactate is generated during muscular work. This lactate diffuses down a twofold gradient into the blood (Diamant, Karlsson, and Saltin, 1968) and is carried to the liver and kidneys, where it is substrate for gluconeogenesis by the Cori cycle (Cori and Cori, 1929). This arrangement illustrates the supportive role of the visceral organs during work. It also suggests that disposition of lactate may be one limit to work capacity. It can be shown that training allows larger work rates with lower levels of lactate production (Margaria, Edwards, and Dill, 1933). Trained men show a

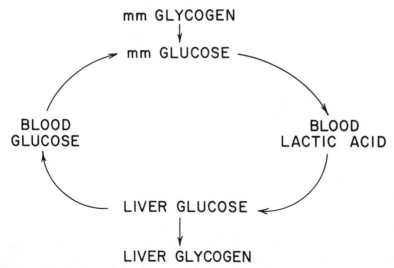

Figure 1. The Cori cycle.

Work supported by the National Live Stock and Meat Board.

quicker reduction to normal of blood lactate levels following the completion of work (Rowell et al., 1966). In several mammals, including man, the rate of lactate production in the resting state is approximately 0.85 mg/kg/min (DePocas, Minaire, and Chatonnet, 1969). During maximal exercise this can be increased at least fivefold. About three-fourths of this lactate is converted to carbon dioxide, and the rest appears as glucose. Only small amounts of lactic acid are excreted in the urine until the blood levels exceed 6 mM/liter (54 mg/100 ml). Holloszy and his associates (1971) have reviewed the evidence for a biochemical adaptation in muscle metabolism with training. There is an increase of mitochondrial protein and an augmentation of several oxidative enzymes. Krebs and his co-workers (1964) have shown with rats that either a low-carbohydrate diet or preliminary exercise will increase the rate of gluconeogenesis in kidney tissue studied in vitro.

The evidence thus suggests that the disposition of lactate generated by exercise is one limit of physical fitness. This hypothesis has three corollaries, which were investigated in this study:

1. The rate of removal of lactate from blood can be augmented by physical training
2. The capacity to remove lactate from blood can be augmented by feeding either L-(+)-lactate or a carbohydrate-free diet
3. The level of physical fitness is correlated with the rate of lactate clearance from the blood, and both fitness and lactate clearance will be augmented by training or by diets that induce the enzymes necessary for lactate clearance through gluconeogenesis.

The evidence collected supported the hypotheses and implied that dietary measures may be used to augment physical fitness.

TESTING EFFECT OF LACTATE
DISPOSITION FROM EXERCISE ON FITNESS

Methods

Mongrel dogs and young adult men in various levels of fitness were used for these studies. Lactate tolerance was measured with a loading dose of sodium L-(+)-lactate given intravenously in 15–30 sec with the subjects in a resting state. The dose was 2 mEq/kg of body weight for dogs and 1.0 mEq/kg body weight for men. The dose differential is necessary to accommodate for the higher removal rate found in dogs. This dose will give blood lactate levels of 30–60 mg/100 ml of whole blood at 8 min after the injection. Blood was drawn at 8, 12, 16, and 20 min and 1 ml was placed immediately in 3 ml of freshly prepared 5% metaphosphoric acid in a weighed tube and mixed by inversion. After

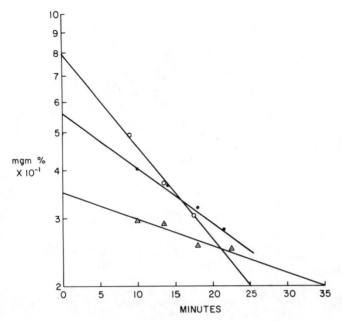

Figure 2. Plots of three lactate tolerance tests showing widely different clearance rates. A computer fit by least squares methods is no improvement on visual fitting. The K_L values are: O=5.41, ●=3.25, and ▲=1.58.

centrifugation, lactate was measured in duplicate in the clear supernatant, using yeast lactic dehydrogenase in the automated method described by Mann and Shute (1970). The decline of blood lactate after 8 min is exponential. The K_L, equivalent to the K_{gl} of glucose tolerance (Mann and Shute, 1970), was calculated. This expresses the percent decline per min of lactate concentration in the blood.

The dogs were trained by treadmill running, using a weighted saddle to increase the work load, and the effect on K_L was measured (Figure 4). Other dogs were fed either a diet of only meat, or a

$$K_L = \frac{(\log_e 2)}{T\frac{1}{2}} \times 100$$

Figure 3. The value for T_{1-2} is obtained from the plot of the log of concentration of lactate with time. Then K_L equals $0.693/T_{1"2} \times 100$.

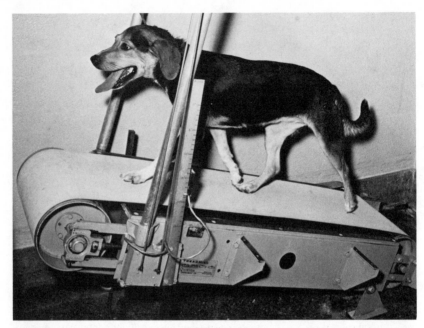

Figure 4. Dogs quickly learn to run on the treadmill. A weighted saddle was used as training progressed to shorten the training times and lessen the grades necessary for training.

carbohydrate-free diet supplemented with L-(1)-lactate (Table 1), which forced them to increase gluconeogenesis.

Results

Serial studies done weekly in untreated dogs and men, yielded the average values for K_L and its variation as shown in Table 2. The average levels of 2.22 ± 0.21 (S.E.M.) for men and 3.07 ± 0.19 (S.E.M.) for dogs are consistent with the higher V_{O_2} max regularly found in dogs (Crescittelli and Taylor, 1944). Training significantly increased the K_L

Table 1.   Composition of a trial diet

Ingredient	Composition (%)
Dry cottage cheese	90
Whole liver powder	1
Calcium lactate (USP)	4
Lactic acid 88%	5
L-lactic acid content	3.92

Table 2. Reproducibility of lactate tolerance test

	Mean	S.E.M.	Coef. variation	S.E. replicate[a]
Human subjects (measured weekly for 9 weeks)				
K_L	2.22	0.21	8.14	0.44
Canine subjects (8 dogs measured weekly for 6 weeks)				
K_L	3.07	0.19	14.1	0.89

$$^a \text{ S.E. Replicate} = \sqrt{\frac{\text{difference of successive determination}^2}{N\text{-}1 \text{ pairs}}}$$

values, as did the COH-free diet (see Figure 5). Because it was difficult to measure fitness accurately in dogs, the work was then applied to men.

The work capacity of human subjects was measured by a Balke type test, in which the men walked on a treadmill at a constant speed of 90 m/min. The grade was increased one angular degree at the end of

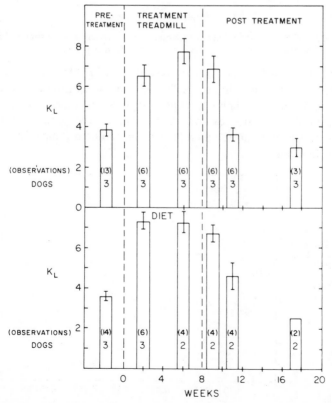

Figure 5. The upper frame shows the effect of training on three dogs with means and S.E.M. The lower frame shows the effect of a CHO-free meat diet on three dogs.

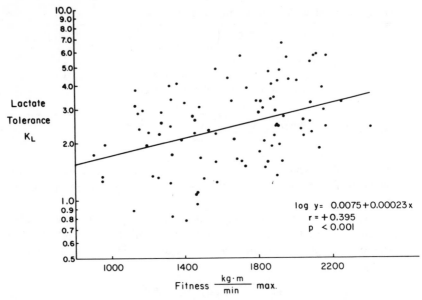

Figure 6. The relation between lactate tolerance expressed as a logarithm and fitness measured as the maximal work capacity in a treadmill test for 96 adult males.

each minute. A pair of electrodes was attached to the chest, and the pulse rate was measured by telemetry. The test was stopped in the first series of experiments when the subject decided he could go no farther. In the second series the test was stopped in a more objective way—when the pulse rate had reached 85% of the predicted maximum for a person of that age.

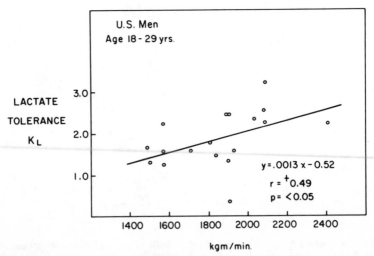

Figure 7. The relationship of K_L and fitness in young men ($N=18$).

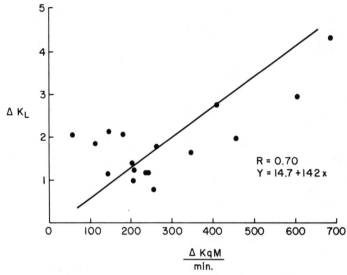

Figure 8. The effect of training on K_L and fitness in young men ($N=17$).

R = 0.70
Y = 14.7 + 142 x

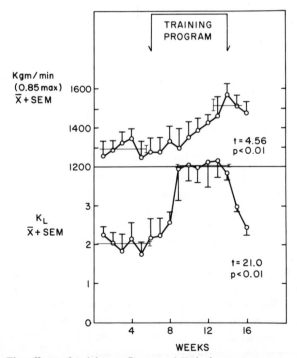

Figure 9. The effects of training on fitness and K_L in four young men.

Paired tests of K_L and fitness (F) in 96 American men, ages 18−55 years, revealed the relationship shown in Figure 6. The correlation is highly significant, although not sufficiently high to be predictive. When 18 men, ages 18−28 years, were considered, in order to diminish a possible confounding effect of age, the correlation coefficient was $r = 0.49$ ($p < 0.05$) (Figure 7).

Seventeen young men were trained 3 to 6 times weekly in 1-hr sessions for periods of 6 to 9 weeks, while both the K_L and F were measured weekly. The increases of the K_L and F were highly correlated (see Figure 8). A similar experiment was repeated with four men who were trained for 9 weeks using the pulse, 85% as the endpoint in the measurement of fitness (Figure 9). Another group of four men was given 5 g of sodium L-(+)-lactate four times daily in Tab, a nonnutritive soft drink manufactured by the Coca-Cola Company. A single dose gave the increase of blood lactate shown in Figure 10. Over a 4-month period, the changes of K_L and F in four male subjects, as shown in Figure 11, were found. Dietary intake of L- lactate alone increased both K_L and F significantly. The experiment was repeated with four men given sodium L-(+)-lactate for four weeks in the same amount and measuring fitness with 85% of expected pulse rate. Again, the same effect was seen.

Discussion

These observations support the hypothesis that one component of fitness is the capacity to dispose of the lactate generated by working muscles. The limit in this process might be the transport of lactate across membranes (Kübler et al., 1965) or some enzymatic step in gluconeogenesis. The identity of the system or enzyme responsible is not presently known. Krebs (1964) has proposed that the limiting enzyme in gluconeogenesis is likely to be at one of four stages of gluconeogenesis (Figure 12): the first involves the conversion of pyruvate to oxaloacetate by pyruvic carboxylase; the second the formation of phosphopyruvate by phosphopyruvatecarboxykinase; the third is the removal of phosphate from fructose 1,6-diphosphate; and the fourth the conversion of glucose 6-phosphate to glucose. Whatever the explanation, the present findings suggest that the rate of clearance of L-(+)-lactate from blood following a standard intravenous dose is correlated with physical fitness and that either training or certain dietary treatments will augment both physical fitness and lactate clearance. Only about half the variance of fitness is accounted for by the change of lactate clearance, so clearance does not accurately predict fitness. The variation of lactate clearance suggests that other factors influence this,

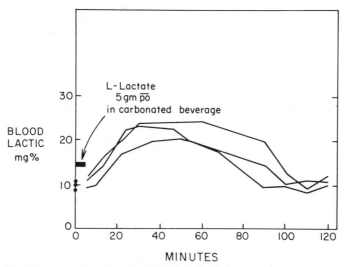

Figure 10. Three men were given 5 g of potassium lactate in 300 ml of Coca Cola over a 1- to 4-min interval. Blood samples were drawn during the following 120 min for L-lactate determination.

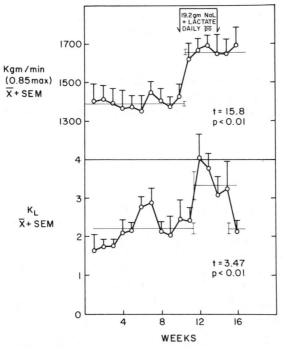

Figure 11. The effects of sodium L-(+)-lactate given in four divided doses to supply 19.2 g daily. Fitness was measured with the objective endpoint of 85% of the predicted maximum pulse rate. The lightly drawn lines show the means before and after treatment from which the t values were calculated.

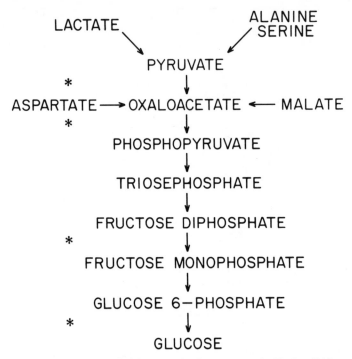

Figure 12. The probable rate limiting steps in gluconeogenesis (Krebs, 1964).

and we have some preliminary evidence that certain common drugs do this. These include ethanol and phenformin. The data do give some insight into the biochemical nature of fitness, and suggest dietary ways of augmenting fitness.

SUMMARY

An intravenous test of lactate clearance from blood was applied to studies of the nature of physical fitness in dogs and men. Both fitness and the rate of clearance of blood lactate were augmented by feeding lactate in man. Training or feeding a carbohydrate-free diet in dogs also augmented lactate clearance in dogs. The present experiments do not indicate whether these effects result from a change in the membrane transport of lactate or by the induction of some limiting enzyme in gluconeogenesis.

REFERENCES

Cori, C. F., and Cori, G. T. 1929. Glycogen formation in the liver from d- and l-lactic acid. J. Biol. Chem. 81: 389.

Crescitelli, F., and Taylor, C. 1944. The lactate response to exercise and its relationship to physical fitness. Amer. J. Physiol. 141: 630.

De Pocas, F., Minaire, Y., and Chatonnet, J. 1969. Rates of formation and oxidation of lactic acid in dogs at rest and during moderate exercise. Canad. J. Physiol. Pharmacol. 47: 603.

Diamant, B., Karlsson, J., and Saltin, B. 1968. Muscle tissue lactate after maximal exercise in man. Act. Physiol. Scand. 72: 383.

Holloszy, J. O., et al. 1971. Biochemical adaptation to endurance exercise in skeletal muscle. In B. Pernow and B. Saltin (eds.), Advances in Experimental Medicine and Biology, Vol. II. Plenum Press, N. Y. 1971.

Krebs, H. 1964. Gluconeogenesis. Proc. Royal Soc. 159: 545.

Kübler, W., et al. 1965 Über du Milchsäure und Brenztraubensäurepermeation aus dem hypothermen Myokard. (Concerning the permeability of lactate and pyroacetic acid through hypothemicmyocardium.) Pflügers Arch. 287: 203.

Mann, G. V., and Shute, E. 1970. An automated method for L-lactate in blood. Clin. Chem. 16: 849.

Margaria, R., Edwards, H. T., and Dill, D. B. 1933. Possible mechanisms of contracting and paying oxygen debt and role of lactic acid in muscular contraction. Amer. J. Physiol. 106: 689.

Rowell, L. B., Kraning, K. K., Evans, H. T. O., Kennedy, J. W., Blackman, J. R., and Kusumi, F. 1966. Splanchnic removal of lactate and pyruvate during prolonged exercise in man. J. Appl. Physiol. 21: 1773.

Carbohydrate Nutrition and Human Performance

J. D. Brooke

Nutritional support from carbohydrate sources and human performance are intimately related. Any textbook of nutrition will identify the long-term requirements of the human for intake of both digestible and indigestible carbohydrates. The present review does not concern itself with these matters of long-term support, but with the effects of varying the amount or types of carbohydrate in the diet upon human performance over a time span not exceeding 2 to 3 weeks. The concern is with research statements that combine information about a) dietary components, b) information about metabolism, possibly central nervous system modifications or responses, and c) subsequent human behavior.

As reviewed in detail in this volume by Saltin, carbohydrate nutrition as support for sustained physical work has been substantially investigated. Information is also now accumulating about its significance for short-term, delicate information processing tasks. However, before surveying this material some additional insight may be helpful.

Following sustained physical work, the effects of nutrition to alter metabolic status are moderated upon by the performance itself. The basis of this alteration is direct utilization of metabolic reservoirs of essential energy. It is, however, becoming clear that the performance act also can have significant *short-term* effects upon metabolic status obtained by prior nutrition. Figure 1 illustrates data from Brooke, Llewelyn, and Green (1976), in which the effects of prior ingestion of glucose syrup solution upon blood glucose levels both at rest and over exercise of 20 min duration at a cycle ergometer work load of 150 W are reported. It should be noted that after ingesting carbohydrate to an energy value of 1.43 MJ, blood glucose values are significantly raised, with the effects of a change in environmental demand and exercise of quite moderate intensity, resulting in marked reversal of that metabolic trend. Simpson, Cox, and Rothschild (1974) reported that short-term skilled performance with prior glucose loading resulted in a marked fall in blood glucose when high noise levels were introduced into the performance environment. It has been noted that when performance is required of a subject, blood glucose response curves to carbohydrate loading reduce demonstrably in comparison to nonperformance conditions. These performance modifications of blood glucose response to carbohydrate ingestion reveal the need for further investigation and for planning in the use of such carbohydrate nutrition, taking into account both the behavioral needs and the appropriate timing of the ingestion. Noting the marked individuality occurring in blood glucose response to such nutrition, there is also the need for sensitive awareness of individual variation. These notes have particular significance in interpreting the studies referred to in this chapter, particularly those pertaining to information processing tasks.

Notwithstanding these constraints, there have been considerable recent advances in describing the very important role of *carbohydrate nutrition in the support of sustained physical work*. With provision of carbohydrate diet, long distance cyclists have ridden further (Brooke, Davies, and Green, 1975), long distance cross country skiers have raced faster (Karlsson and Saltin, 1971), long distance canoeists have

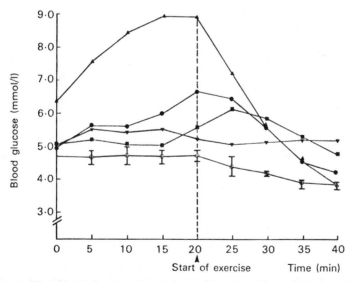

Figure 1. Mean blood glucose values in four adult male subjects during exercise after ingestion of glucose syrup (G): ○, G not given; ▼, G given at start of exercise; ■, G given 10 min before exercise; ●, G given 20 min before exercise; ▲, G given 30 min before exercise. Vertical bars indicate standard deviations of mean values for four subjects. (Reproduced by permission of Cambridge University Press from Brooke, J. D., Llewelyn K., and Green, L. F. *Proc. Nutr. Soc.* 1976. 35. 136A.)

paddled faster (Green and Bagley, 1972), and soccer players have scored more goals in the latter part of matches (Muckle, 1973). The basis for many of these reported effects from the field is firmly established in metabolic physiology (see Saltin, this volume). It seems that availability of carbohydrate is a major limiting factor and that digestible dietary carbohydrate taken during the performance or utilized in conjunction with prior exercise or used to facilitate recovery plays an important role. For reasons that are not at present clear, the other available energy substrate, fat, does not seem to be available to maintain performance at intensities of 60 to 75% Vo_2 max. Neither the supply of free fatty acids exogenous to the active muscle (Zierler et al., 1968) nor the endogenously available muscle triglyceride (Carlson, Ekelund, and Fröberg, 1977) can fully replace the essential role of carbohydrates. Thus, carbohydrate nutrition holds a central position for such performance. It should be noted that no increase in urinary nitrogen excretion is seen with physical acitivity, which suggests that in normally fed subjects, protein does not usually contribute additional energy for the maintenance of physical work, and thus attention toward nutrients for such performances has been directed instead to the fats and carbohydrates.

In comparison to such studies of sustained demanding work, some study has been made of the role of carbohydrate metabolism for maximum short-term physical work tasks. Taylor, Lappage, and Rao (1977) did not find a decrement in muscle glycogen stores following maximum short-term physical work on a cycle ergometer. This may be interpreted to indicate that such stores were not acting as a limit to that type of performance. With reference to short-term swimming performances, Haldi and Wynn (1946) found no effect upon performance of eating heavy or light meals 2 to 3 hr before performance, nor did they find any effect from supplementation of the diet with 50 or 100 g of sucrose immediately before performance.

In considering the role of carbohydrate nutrition in vigorous physical work, it is appropriate to take cognizance of the need for dietary carbohydrates when accidental hypothermia or exposure is imminent because of accidents on outdoor expeditions. Taylor (1972), Campbell (1972), and Berkeley (1973) draw attention to the interaction of hypoglycemia with hypothermia in cases of exposure and cold survival. As reported by Parker and George (1975), shivering thermogenesis markedly depletes metabolic carbohydrate, and in conjunction with meal omission and physical work depletion of local and perhaps more central energy stores, it has much potential to reduce blood glucose levels to fasting and subfasting conditions. Planning to make carbohydrate nutrition available to meet such emergencies is essential.

In the discussion of the topic of survival, a methodological note is of importance with regard to the conduct of studies investigating the role of carbohydrates in sustained physical work tasks or the translation of such studies into field practices in sports, armed forces, industrial, and expedition applications. It became apparent some time ago in the author's own laboratory that subjects well habituated to withstand the pain and distress of the developing anaerobiosis that characterizes short-term physical work exertion were capable of transferring such tolerance to studies where initial hypoglycemia and lack of availability of carbohydrate characterized exhaustion. The result in some situations was symptoms of advancing hypoglycemia. Therefore, it is suggested that a cut-off point be determined beyond which subjects will not be allowed to continue even though they do not perceive themselves as completely exhausted. In some of the initial work this cut-off point was a respiratory quotient of 0.75 to 0.73.

Furthermore, when subjects ingest substantial amounts of carbohydrate in order to carry out high levels of physical activity over hours, it is important to attend to the thiamine, riboflavin, and niacin intakes of the performers. The World Health Organization (1967) noted that for these particular vitamins minimum daily requirements were based on the average energy expenditure. Where energy expenditure is markedly elevated, the daily B vitamin intake also should be elevated. The World Health Organization's "normal" recommendation is 0.9 mg thiamine per 10.0 MJ energy ingested, 1.3 mg riboflavin per 10.0 MJ energy ingested, and 15.7 niacin equivalents per 10.0 MJ energy ingested. In this context, attention is directed to Zaburkin and Minkh (1972), who report that in rats swimming 3 hr daily and also in physical education students taking much exercise, daily modification of the B vitamin complex intake resulted in improvements in physical work capacity. It is worthy of note that the B_1 vitamin, thiamine, is substantially lost through the cooking process, as is vitamin C. Most nutrients are extremely stable, even the vitamins, but vitamin B_1 does suffer from leaching from food, and is particularly unstable in neutral and alkaline pH conditions. It is easily oxidized, is destroyed by sulphur dioxide, and there is marked loss through heating.

As well as attending to relationships with sustained physical work, researchers of carbohydrate nutrition in human performance have also attended to *tasks where information processing and subsequent response,* in comparison to the generation of physical work, are the main characteristics. In this domain, a number of studies concerned particularly with the provision or omission of meals and subsequent performance were conducted in the period before 1950 and are reviewed in Brooke (1973). In some instances interpretation of the studies is difficult, because of the advances that have been made in experimental control in recent years. A number of recent studies report results suggesting or indicating a relationship between level of blood glucose and fine skilled performance. Fraser, Buck, and McKendry (1974) reported that in 50% of subjects given intravenous injections of insulin to lower blood glucose, response execution on a tracking task was significantly impaired in comparison to intravenous injection of saline control. However, there were no changes in the accuracy of final performance, despite the fact that the seven affected subjects showed clear clinical signs of hypoglycemia in conjunction with plasma glucose concentrations of 1.76 mmole/liter or less. The impairment lasted from the 15th to the 60th min following injection. This study clearly obtruded deeply into clinical conditions. In comparison, Simpson, Cox, and Rothschild (1974), through ingestion of 18 g of glucose in 100 ml of water by 3-hr fasting subjects, demonstrated alleviation of performance impairment induced by 80 dB(A) white noise intruded into the environment of a pursuit rotor tracking task. The glucose-fed group, when not under sound stressor, also showed a much shallower fall in blood glucose level back toward normal values during the test. However, in the no-noise condition, glucose ingestion resulted in a fall in tracking performance. Brooke et al. (1973) reported a relationship between reduction in factory accidents and intake of glucose syrup drink (Birch, Green, and Coulson, 1970) to elevate worker's low respiratory quotients and blood glucose levels because of breakfast omission. Such studies suggest that ingestion of carbohydrate has an impact upon more delicate types of human performance.

This conclusion is supported by a number of more peripheral observations. Levine, Gordon, and Derick (1924) reported that marathon runners with low blood glucose levels exhibited emotional changes, Christensen and Hansen (1939) reported perceptual disturbances in subjects with low blood glucose levels during the physical work research reported above, and also, as previously reported, perceptual disturbances occurred in subjects in the author's own laboratories near the end of such physical work trials. Harris (1933) has reported that signs of hypoglycemia appear for some subjects as they pass below the fasting level of 4.1 mmole/liter blood glucose, and Keele and Niel (1971) also denote this boundary position. Because blood glucose levels in the range of 3.3 mmole/liter are common in studies of sustained demanding physical work, and indeed Ahlborg et al. (1967) report values of 2.5 and 2.7 mmole/liter, such changes might be expected and could be anticipated to intrude into the total skill performance capacity of humans at such times. In this context, a set of letters to the Editor of the British Medical Journal in 1972 drew attention to low blood glucose levels implicated in motorway accidents (Frais 1972; Leyshon et al., 1972), and Christian (1972) supplied supporting data from a hospital accident unit adjacent to one of the major British motorways.

Such studies may be related to those of extended work, because altered information-processing capability has been involved at times in such research to account for effects not seen as of local metabolic causation. Christensen and Hansen (1939) reported that subjects exhausted by extended work and then fed glucose could continue work for an additional hour, although indications of metabolic fuel from the respiratory quotient were unaltered from the exhausted state. Blood glucose values were elevated. Brooke and Green (1974) noted similar effects when a second bout of work following 40 min rest and carbohydrate feeding was required in comparison to feeding with high fat/high carbohydrate diets, or with no feeding. Åstrand (1967) has suggested there may be a neural basis for the phenomenon, implying a change in signaling function. Furthermore, maintenance of efficiency of work beyond that expected from the associated metabolic data in extended industrial and in laboratory work under carbohydrate dietary treatments has been reported by Benade et al. (1973) and Brooke, Davies, and Green (1975).

It is pertinent to question the basis for effects on information processing. At present, a number of hypotheses can be advanced. It is possible that the level of the blood glucose is either a determining or potentiating factor, and two mechanisms already have support available. First, it might be considered that lowered glucose levels below the typical fasting value act to challenge directly the metabolism of nerve cells. Although studies on central nervous system metabolism (Owen et al., 1967) have shown that up to 60% of resting CNS energy requirements can be met by ketone bodies in the human, this still leaves 40% of the energy demand as essential glucose. Indeed, evaluation of brain arteriovenous gas differences indicates that approximately 93% of cellular energy is normally derived from carbohydrate. These were the findings that earlier led researchers to conclude that the central nervous system depended solely on glucose for metabolism. It is clear now that this is not the case, but it is also clear that there is an essential need for glucose, and it may be that in the studies already reported here, this essential need is not being completely met. In this context, it is interesting to note that in sustained demanding physical work studies, it is common to see the blood glucose level of unfed subjects move quickly to a fasting value and then to hold at that value, comparatively stable over the succeeding hours, while the RQ gradually falls, indicating increased dependence on the fat contribution to the metabolic mixture.

Because the blood glucose reservoir is only very slowly depleted in such conditions, there is the implication that it is important for the integrity of the whole organism that the fasting value be supported. The difficulty in evaluating such proposals lies in the marked interindividual variability in susceptibility to the onset of hypoglycemic symptoms. If glucose provision for metabolism of nerve cell is hypothesized to be the effect resulting in performance deterioration, account should also be taken of the other side of the metabolic equation at such times, i. e., that a component of the increasing fat metabolism might be the disruptive factor.

In reference to the level of the blood glucose, recent work by Wurtman and Fernstrom (1974) has led to the proposal of an alternate hypothesis. This research has indicated that with appropriate levels of circulating neutral amino acids, ingestion of carbohydrates to elevate blood glucose levels results in a metabolic chain being triggered by the increased insulin release, resulting eventually in increased levels of the central nervous transmitter substance 5-hydroxytryptamine. Because clinical pharmaceutical intervention to elevate this transmitter is associated with relief of depression and change in mood, it is possible that carbohydrate ingestion in the fine skill tasks described above is acting to modify performance through modification of this CNS synaptic agent.

With regard to the integration of neural function, a further hypothesis that cannot be discounted is that feelings of distress from fasting conditions are competing, at central nervous levels associated with perceptual selection, for central attentive space (Moray, 1969). It is clear from studies of attention and the ascending reticular activating system that feelings of discomfort or pain markedly distort the perceptual field, and this effect cannot be discounted for the present situations. These competing hypotheses remain undifferentiated to date.

A recent study from the author's laboratories provides preliminary information concerning changes in nerve function associated with decreased carbohydrate availability (Brooke, in press). Subjects carried out sustained physical work trials over hours to exhaustion of available carbohydrate stores, and 20 min pre- and post-work were tested for reaction time and its components (premotor and motor time) by EMG recordings. On some trials subjects were unfed throughout the trial, on other trials they were fed a glucose syrup solution or low energy control drink every 20 min during work, and on some trials subjects were fed glucose syrup solution immediately at the end of work. Some subjects showed marked deterioration in reaction time or its components in the unfed condition, and for some of these subjects, this was alleviated wholly or partially as a result of carbohydrate ingestion. However, note was made of the marked individual variability between subjects, with some subjects showing no effect at all as a result of the carbohydrate depletion or the carbohydrate nutrition. Post-work blood glucose levels did not account for this variability, and it requires further study.

Guetzkow et al. (1945) carried out similar measurements on resting subjects, and reported a significant correlation between level of blood glucose and reaction time when the blood glucose was below the level of 3.6−3.8 mmole/liter. Reaction time and blood glucose were not related above this level. It is possible that the same interpretation can be placed upon the report by Muckle (1973) that ingestion of glucose syrup solution during 20 professional soccer matches improved both team and individual performance, assessed by goals scored and conceded, the total number of scoring efforts, and ball contacts.

From the studies that have been reviewed, it seems that there is need to pay attention to normal human carbohydrate nutrition and variations in skilled performance. Evaluation of this position is complicated by the amount of inter- and intrasubject variation that occurs in both level of blood glucose with a standard carbohydrate challenge and in the incidence of performance deterioration or hypoglycemic symptoms as a function of blood glucose level. These added complexities are well illustrated by the problems associated with the reproducibility and interpretation of the standard clinical glucose tolerance test. Butterfield (1964) observed that no clear segregation of blood glucose values into two populations could be observed in a study of 24,701 subjects, but that there was a smooth gradation of values. Thus, the criteria for diagnosis of diabetes was felt to be somewhat arbitrary. Reporting later in the same paper on further tests on a random sample of 27,000 people, the author noted, "all of us are glycaemic, some are more glycaemic than others" (p. 199). Danowski (1963, p. 446) came to a similar conclusion, as did Roberts (1964), identifying a "twilight biochemical zone," within which it was difficult to differentiate normal from clinically diabetic populations. Such zones command research from the biologist studying normal humans. However, careful control of confounding variables is required. McDonald, Fisher, and Burnham (1965) noted that in a standard glucose tolerance test, it is common for a subject to vary peak blood glucose values by as much as ± 1.9 mmole/liter from test to test, and both Roberts (1964) and Jarrett et al. (1972) have reported diurnal variation in oral glucose tolerance. Additionally, Jarrett and Graver (1968) noted variability in oral glucose tolerance during the menstrual cycle. It is clear that a number of factors have an impact upon metabolic condition resulting from carbohydrate ingestion. Some of these factors are performance characteristics, others include individual variations introduced through such variables as emotional status and biological rhythm. Laboratory research attending to the fine motor part of the task domain needs to control such potentially confounding variables.

Accordingly, when turning to field applications of the present research, great care needs to be taken. It is clear that the maintenance of blood glucose is significantly related to the incidence of meal frequency (Thornton and Horvath, 1968), and Fàbry (1969) substantially reviews the interrelation between feeding pattern, metabolic effects, and performance in the field. However, as the Office of Health Economics, London (1969) pointed out:

> At this stage much research is needed to assess . . . whether such non-specific symptoms as loss of appetite, general malaise, insomnia, increased irritability can be and on occasions are the result of nutritional problems (p.21).

When precision of performance and error or accidents are added to the above list, the directive continues to carry weight today. With the gradual accumulation of empirical studies in closely related areas, there is now further need to study in the normal human being the relationship between carbohydrate ingestion, metabolic status, nervous system integration, and skilled performance.

REFERENCES

Ahlborg, B., Bergström, J., Ekelund, L. F., and Hultman, E. 1967. Muscle glycogen and muscle electrolytes during prolonged physical exercise. Acta. Physiol. Scand. 70: 129—142.

Åstrand, P. O. 1967. Diet and athletic performance. Fed. Proc. 26: 1772—7.

Benade, A. J. S., Wyndham, C. H., Jansen, C. R., Rogers, G. G., and Bruin, E. J. P. 1973. Plasma insulin and carbohydrate metabolism after sucrose ingestion during rest and prolonged aerobic exercise. Pflugers Archiv. 342: 207—218.

Birch, G. G., Green, L. F., and Coulson, C. B. 1970. Glucose syrups and related carbohydrates. Elsevier, London.

Brooke, J. D. 1973. Carbohydrates and human performance. In G.G. Birch and L.F. Green (eds.), Molecular Structure and Function of Food Carbohydrates. Applied Sciences, London.

Brooke, J. D. Effects on fractionated reaction time of sustained movement to deplete metabolic carbohydrate. Proc. Int. Congr. Phys. Act. Sci. Quebec. In press.

Brooke, J. D., Davies, G. J., and Green, L. F. 1975. The effects of normal and glucose syrup work diets on the performance of racing cyclists. J. Sports Med. Phys. Fitness 15(3): 257—265.

Brooke, J. D., and Green, L. F. 1974. The effect of a high carbohydrate diet on human recovery following prolonged work to exhaustion. Ergonomics 17(4): 489—497.

Brooke, J. D., and Green, L. F. 1976. Effect of close and open spaced work trials upon endurance and body carbohydrate stores in trained endurance sportsmen. J. Sports Med. Phys. Fitness 15(2): 91–99.

Brooke, J. D., Llewelyn, K., and Green, L. F. 1976. Time of glucose syrup ingestion to alleviate initial exercise hypoglycaemia. Proc. Nutr. Soc. 35: 136A.

Brooke, J. D., Toogood, S., Green, L. F., and Bagley, R. 1973. Factory accidents and carbohydrate supplements. Proc. Nutr. Soc. 32: 94A.

Butterfield, W. J. H. 1964. Bedford diabetes survey. Proc. R. Soc. Med. 57: 196–200.

Campbell, I. A. 1972. Mountain accidents. Br. J. Sports Med. 6(3,4): 108–110.

Carlson, L. A., Ekelund, L., and Fröberg, S. O. 1977. Concentration of triglycerides, phospholipids and glycogen in skeletal muscle and of free fatty acids and beta—hydroxybutyric acid in blood in man in response to exercise. Europ. J. Clin. Invest. 1: 248–254.

Christensen, E. H., and Hansen, O. 1939. Arbeitsfähigkeit und Ernähung. Scand. Arch. Physiol. 81: 160–172.

Christian, M. S. 1972. Letter to the Editor—Multiple crashes on motorways. Br. Med. J. 29 April.

Danowski, T. W. 1963. Emotional stress as a cause of diabetes mellitus. Diabetes 12: 183.

Fàbry, P. 1969. Feeding Pattern and Nutritional Adaptions. Butterworth, London.

Frais, J. A. 1972. Letter to the Editor—Multiple crashes on motorways. Br. Med. J. 1 April.

Fraser, B. A., Buck, L., and McKendry, J. B. R. 1974. Psychomotor performance during insulin-induced hypoglycaemia. Can. Med. Assoc. J. 110: 513–518.

Green, L. F., and Bagley, R. 1972. Ingestion of a glucose syrup drink during long distance canoeing. Br. J. Sports Med. 6(3,4): 125–128.

Guetzkow, H., Taylor, H. L., Brozek, J., and Keys, A. 1945. Relationship of speed of motor reaction to blood sugar level during acute starvation in man. Fed. Proc. 4: 28.

Haldi, J., and Wynn, W. 1946. The effect of low and high carbohydrate meals on the blood sugar level and on work performance in strenuous exercise of short duration. Am. J. Physiol. 145: 402.

Harris, S. 1933. Hyperinsulinism, a definite disease entity. J. Am. Med. Assoc. 101:1958.

Jarrett, R. J., and Graver, H. J. 1968. Changes in oral glucose tolerance during the menstrual cycle. Br. Med. J. 2: 528–529.

Jarrett, R. J., Baker, I. A., Keen, H., and Oakly, N. W. 1972. Diurnal variation in oral glucose tolerance: Blood sugar and plasma insulin levels morning, afternoon and evening. Br. Med. J. 1 (5794): 199–201.

Karlsson, J., and Saltin, B. 1971. Diet, muscle glycogen and endurance performance. J. Appl. Physiol. 31(2): 203–206.

Keele, C. A., and Neil, E. 1971. Sampson Wright's Applied Physiology. 12th ed. Oxford, London.

Levine, S. A., Gordon, B., and Derick, C. L. 1924. J. Am. Med. Assoc. 81: 1778.

Leyshon, G. F., Elliott, R. W., Lyons, J., and Francis, H. W. S. 1972. Letter to the Editor—Diabetics and motorway accidents. Br. Med. J. 12 May.

McDonald, G. W., Fisher, G. F., and Burnham, C. 1965. Reproducibility of the oral glucose tolerance test. Diabetes 14: 473–480.

Moray, N. 1969. Attention: Selective Processes in Vision and Hearing. Hutchinson, London.

Muckle, D. S. 1973. Glucose syrup ingestion and team performance in soccer. Br. J. Sports Med. 7(364): 340–343.

Office of Health Economics. 1969. Malnutrition in the 1960's. HMSO, London.

Owen, O. E., Morgan, A. P., Kemp, H. G., Sullivan, J. M., Herrera, M. G., and Cahil, C. G. 1967. Brain metabolism during fasting. J. Clin. Invest. 46(10): 1589–1595.

Parker, G. H., and George, J. C. 1975. Effects of short and long term exercise on intracellular glycogen and fat in pigeon pectoralis. Japan. J. Physiol. 25: 175–184.

Roberts, H. J. 1964. Afternoon glucose testing. J. Am. Geriatr. Soc. 12: 423.

Simpson, G. C., Cox, T., and Rothschild, D. R. 1974. The effects of noise stress on blood glucose level and skilled performance. Ergonomics 17(4): 481–487.

Taylor, A. W., Lappage, R., and Rao, S. 1977. Skeletal muscle glycogen stores after submaximal and maximal work. Med. Sci. Ex. Sports 3(2): 75–78.

Taylor, D. E. M. 1972. Cold survival. Br. J. Sports Med. 6(3,4): 111–116.

Thornton, R. H., and Horvath, S. M. 1968. Blood glucose as influenced by either one or two meals. J. Am. Diet. Assoc. 52: 214–217.

World Health Organization. 1967. Expert group in requirements of vitamin A, thiamine, riboflavine and niacin. WHO Techn. Rep. Ser. No. 362.

Wurtman, R. J., and Fernstrom, J. D. 1974. Effects of the diet on brain transmitters. Nutr. Rev. 32(7): 193–200.

Zaburkin, E. M., and Minkh, A. A. 1972. Changes in some values of pyridoxine and nicotinic acid metabolism during physical stress. Vestn. Akad. Med. Nauk SSSR 1: 60–65.

Zierler, K. L., Moseri, A., Klassen, G., Rubinowitz, D., and Burgess, J. 1968. Trans. Assoc. Am. Physicians 81: 266.

Protein Requirements and Physical Activity

J. V. G. A. Durnin

For most European and American populations, there is an abundance of dietary information to show that, for a majority of people, at least 10–12% of the total energy of their food comes from protein. With total energy intakes varying from 2,000 to 4,000 kcal/day, this means a protein intake of 50 to 120 g/day.

The main concern of this chapter is whether or not an individual undertaking hard physical activity whose intake falls within this range will always be receiving enough protein. Is a higher protein intake beneficial?

There has existed, possibly for hundreds of years, a widespread belief that violent muscular exercise requires the eating of a large amount of meat. In the first half of the last century, Von Liebig (1842) gave scientific support to this presumption by proposing that during exercise the substance of the muscles is used up, and that protein is the fuel of muscular work. In Britain, at about the same time, the surveys of Playfair (1865), Professor of Chemistry in Edinburgh, seemed to reinforce this view; from his findings that hard-working laborers had high intakes of protein in their diet he set down protein requirements ranging from 57 g/day for a subsistence diet to 184 g/day for heavy laborers.

At the anecdotal level, Drummond and Wilbraham (1939), in their history of the Englishman's diet over five centuries, described how the Oxford rowing crew in the 1860s trained on a diet consisting only of meat, bread, tea, and beer. Throughout the 1860s they consistently defeated the Cambridge boat crew, whose diet was very varied and included potatoes, green vegetables, and fruit—clearly, protein seemed more effective than vitamins!

Voit (1881) lent his distinguished reputation to the concept of the desirability of a high protein content in the diet, and concluded that an average working man should receive 118 g protein daily, 56 g of fat, and 500 g of carbohydrate. For heavy workers, higher intakes were considered necessary.

Much later, the German physiologist Rubner, a most eminent nutritionist, propounded the view that a large amount of protein in the diet promoted the vigor and physical efficiency of the physically active man. During the first World War he had considerable influence on food policy in Germany, and he encouraged German agriculture in its policy of rearing cattle and sheep at the expense of cereals. His ignorance of the fact that cereals can yield several times more dietary energy per acre than meat production significantly worsened the severe effects of food shortage in Germany in 1917, following the blockade by the Allied fleets of food imports.

Opposing viewpoints to the idea that large protein intakes are necessary for optimal physical work have an almost equally long history. Although Voit accepted the view of Liebig that protein was the source of muscular energy, experiments with his collaborator Pettenkofer (Pettenkofer and Voit, 1866) showed that exercise was not associated with a significant increase in nitrogen excretion. At this time too, Fick and Wislicenus (1865) performed their historic climb to the top of the Faulhorn, which demonstrated that protein was *not* the fuel for muscular work. In the early years of this century, the American physiologist Chittenden (1909), in experiments lasting many months on himself and on soldiers and athletes with protein intakes of usually no more than 50–55 g/day, and sometimes as little as 40 g/day, concluded that such low intakes were not only compatible with health and physical performance, but were even beneficial. He claimed that the extra work of excreting N from the high protein diet throws a strain on the kidneys and tends to cause renal and vascular disease. There is little to support his idea of renal damage resulting from large amounts of N excretion, because several small populations—e.g., the Gaucho of the South American plains and the Masai of Central Africa—may have protein intakes of 250 to 300 g daily, and seem to tolerate these well.

On the other hand, the well-known animal studies of McCay and his co-workers (McCay, Crowell, and Maynard, 1935; McCay et al., 1939) demonstrated that serious restriction of energy and protein intakes enabled the animals to live longer and to be physiologically younger at any age. Holt, Halac, and Kajdi (1962) presented good evidence to show that laboratory rats kept on low protein diets, allowing no reserve of protein to accumulate, resist stresses such as exercise, unfavorable environmental temperatures, and even infections and injuries, as well as rats provided with an excess of protein.

It would be better, of course, to have such well-controlled observations on human beings as well as on laboratory animals, but studies on man are often much less meticulously carried out and are less convincing. However, one way or another, the cumulative evidence on man makes it difficult to believe that there are significant increases in protein requirements caused by heavy physical exercise. There are the older studies of Thomas (1910), Zuntz (1911), and Cathcart and Burnett (1926). There is the more recent work of Margaria and Foa (1939), who observed no change in nitrogen excretion with a change from resting to work situations. Kraut and Lehmann (1948) found no differences in the amount of dietary protein required for nitrogen balance during several months of studying miners at rest and at work. Nöcker (1951) found no increase in nitrogen excretion as a result of a 20 km march. There may be small increases in N losses with exercise (Cathcart, 1921) (perhaps of the order of 1 g N/day—equivalent to about 6 g protein), but it has been suggested (Wilson, 1932; Blaxter, 1963) that even this is not a result of the exercise but of accelerated protein metabolism resulting from the higher protein intakes in the diet.

The timing of exercise in relation to meals is related to this and is of importance, and Cuthbertson, McGirr, and Munro (1937) found that N losses were greater when work was performed soon after a meal compared to physical activity in the post-absorptive period. This may be attributable to the fact that there is an impairment in the normal deposition of amino acids in muscle that occurs shortly after a meal, because of the physical activity of the muscles.

Perhaps, having reviewed the classical literature and having looked at the standard textbooks where, almost without exception, every reputable book of biochemistry, physiology, or nutrition would be unanimous and emphatic in saying that extra protein in the diet is unnecessary for muscular exercise, we yet have niggling doubts about the universality of that proposition. We can still examine the problem in a more basic way.

How, and in what quantities, is protein (or, as it is measured, N) lost from the body? There are several routes of loss:

1. There is always a certain amount excreted in the urine because of the endogenous metabolism of protein, the protein turnover that occurs continuously in the tissues. This has not been shown to increase as a result of exercise, other than the very small amounts reported by Cathcart. Although there is individual variability in urinary N excretion, the mean estimate for men is about 37 mg N/kg body weight (FAO/WHO, 1973). The equivalent value for women might be expected to be less, because of the lower relative fat-free mass, but the experimental data show little difference (Murlin et al., 1946).

2. There is also a loss of N in the feces, even when no protein is being consumed, presumably because of loss of cells and secretions from

the intestinal tract. There is no suggestion that exercise has an influence here. Again, there is a considerable range for normal adult men, but the mean value is about 12 mg of N/kg of body weight.

3. Losses occur from the skin in the form of desquamated cells, hair, nails, and in sweat, and this amounts to about 5 mg of N/kg of body weight for men. Although Consolazio et al. (1966) found large losses of N in the sweat of soldiers exposed for short periods to high environmental temperatures, these have not been described for people accustomed to living and working in hot climates. In a tropical climate skin losses of N are probably about twice as great as those in a temperate environment (10 mg N/kg as opposed to 5 mg N/kg).

Sweating as a result of vigorous physical activity increases N loss, and this may amount to a total of about 600 mg in a 2-hr period of strenuous exercise. If this level of activity lasted for 4 hr in the day, entailing an expenditure of 2,400 kcal, the N loss in the sweat would be 1.2 g, requiring an extra 7.5 g of protein to replace this—not a very large amount!

Table 1 shows that the total N losses via the *urine, feces,* and *skin* use about 56 mg N/kg body weight, or about 3.9 g N for a 70 kg man—equivalent to 25 g of protein. This is an average value for a population of men, and does not allow for individual variability. From the published work, the extent of this variability has a coefficient of variation of 15%, so that an addition of twice this amount, 30%, should encompass 97.5% of the population. This means a protein intake of 25 g + 30%, or 32.5 g. Allowing for 4 hr of strenuous exercise with consequent *sweat* losses of N, an addition of a further 7.5 g of protein is required, leading to a grand total of 40 g of protein daily for a 70 kg

Table 1.   Obligatory losses of nitrogen of adult men

	mg N per kg of body weight	
Urine	37	
Feces	12	
Skin	5	
(sweating)		(600 to 1,200 mg total)
Miscellaneous	2	
Total	56	(plus sweat losses)
	Total N losses for a 70 kg man = 3.92 g	
	Equivalent protein = 3.92 × 6.25 = *24.5 g*	

Table 2.   Protein intakes at varying levels of energy intake

Body weight (kg)	Energy intake (kcal/day)	Energy from protein (kcal/day) 10%	15%	Protein intake (g/day) 10%	15%	(g/kg/day) 10%	15%	Requirement (g/kg/day)
80	5,000	500	750	125	187	1.6	2.3	
								0.6
	6,000	600	900	150	225	1.9	2.8	
70	3,000	300	450	75	113	1.1	1.6	

man. These are not very different from the intakes found in certain populations of physically active, muscularly well developed people (cf. the studies of Norgan, Ferro-Luzzi, and Durnin, 1974, on New Guineans).

If *muscle mass* is being markedly increased, a further allowance of 1,000 mg N would include almost every conceivable extreme circumstance for athletes, thus adding another 6−7 g of protein to the requirements—but *only* during the phase of active muscle building. The total now becomes 47 g protein per day.

Let us now examine total intakes of energy and protein by athletes in a variety of circumstances where physical activity is required. In Poland, Celejowa (1973) reported energy intakes of between 5,000 and 6,000 kcal/day in Polish weight lifters. On such diets the protein content would almost certainly vary from about 10% of the total energy, at the lowest level, to 15% or more at the upper end of the scale. Table 2 shows the resultant protein intakes, as g/day and g/kg of body weight/day. For the weight lifters the intakes vary from about 1.1 to 2.8 g/kg/day, compared to an estimated requirement of about 0.6 g/kg/day. It is theoretically inconceivable that such intakes are anything other than grossly in excess of the most extravagant assessment of requirement.

At energy intakes of half these quoted values—that is, at around 3,000 kcal/day, which would be modest levels for the supposed energy outputs of most athletes and men working in heavy occupations—the equivalent intakes of protein vary from 1.1 g/kg/day to 1.6 g/kg/day, and are still two to three times more than estimated requirements. The apparent adequacy of such diets is reinforced by the experiment of Consolazio et al. (1975) on two groups of men consuming 1.4 and 2.8 g protein/kg body weight/day. The men on the higher protein intake had small increases in body protein stores and in muscle mass but showed no improvement in the physiological performance of the work.

What then is the significance of the studies showing some contrary results? Yamaji (1951a,b) observed that increasing the protein intake from 1–1.5 g/kg to 2 g or more per kg body weight resulted in a higher "protein reserve" and a smaller reduction in hemoglobin and serum albumin levels at the beginning of a period of heavy physical training. Yoshimura (1970) similarly showed that the fall in hemoglobin and serum protein could be prevented by high protein intakes (2.5 g/kg body weight). Costill (1976) has pointed out possible misinterpretations of these results. He suggests that there is no real fall in Hb or plasma protein *mass,* because it is the temporary increase in plasma volume resulting from exercise that produces the fall in Hb and plasma protein *concentration.* Stucke et al. (1972), in a study on 20 male athletes on "normal" and high (2 g/kg) protein intakes, found that extra protein significantly increased body weight, the dimensions of the upper arms and thighs (because of thickening of the muscle fibers), the total serum protein, red cell count, and hemoglobin, and lowered the pulse rate in exercise—a remarkable series of findings, some at least of which must be acute changes and cast some doubt on the control exerted over the initial state of the athletes!

Information giving both sides has been presented in this chapter. The general weight of all the scientific data seems to point in one direction. The only valid conclusion to the evidence seems to be that the normal diets of almost all athletes are bound to supply enough protein—theoretically. The theory is amply supported by a great variety of experiments carried out over more than 100 years. Therefore, before reports are accepted that prove the contrary, they need to have been meticulously controlled and carried out, and the results require careful examination. The evidence causes skepticism about any requirement of protein of much more than 1 g/kg body weight/day—which will almost always be supplied by an athlete's diet.

REFERENCES

Blaxter, K. L. 1963. Protein metabolism and requirements in pregnancy and lactation. In H.N. Munro and Allison (eds.), Mammalian Protein Metabolism, Vol. II, pp. 173–223. Academic Press, London.

Cathcart, E. P. 1921. The Physiology of Protein Metabolism. Longmans, Green, London.

Cathcart, E. P., and Burnett, W. A. 1926. The influence of muscle work on metabolism in varying conditions of diet. Proc. R. Soc. Brit. 99: 405–426.

Celejowa, I. 1973. The energy balance in Polish weight-lifters during training in camps from 1961 to 1967. In Physical Fitness, pp. 104–112. Prague.

Chittenden, R. H. 1909. The Nutrition of Man. Heinemann, London.

Consolazio, C. F., Johnson, H. L., Nelson, R. Q., Dramise, J. G., and Skala, J. H. 1975. Protein metabolism of intensive physical training in the young adult. Amer. J. Clin. Nutr. 28: 29–35.

Consolazio, C. F., Matoush, L. O., Nelson, R. A., Isaac, G. J., and Canham, J. E. 1966. Comparisons of nitrogen, calcium and iodine excretion in arm and total body sweat. Amer. J. Clin. Nutr. 18: 443–448.

Costill, D. L. 1976. Muscle water and electrolytes of acute and repeated bouts of dehydration. In International Symposium on Athlete Nutrition, pp. 123–143. Polish Sports Federation, Warsaw.

Cuthbertson, D. P., McGirr, J. L., and Munro, H. N. 1937. A study of the effect of overfeeding on the protein metabolism of man, the effect of muscular work at different levels of energy intake with particular reference to the timing of the work in relation to the taking of food. Biochem. J. 31: 2293–2305.

Drummond, J. C., and Wilbraham, A. 1939. The Englishman's Food. Jonathan Cape, London.

FAO/WHO. 1973. Energy and protein requirements. Report of a joint Ad Hoc Expert Committee. Serial no. 522, pp. 5–118.

Fick, A., and Wislicenus, J. 1865. On the origin of muscular power. Phil. Mag. 31: 485–503.

Holt, L. E., Halac, E., and Kajdi, C. N. 1962. The concept of protein stores and its implications in diet. J. Am. Med. Assoc. 181: 699–705.

Kraut, H., and Lehmann, G. 1948. Der Eiweissbedarf des Schuerarbeiters. (The protein needs of manual workers.) Biochem. Z. 319: 228–246.

McCay, C. M., Crowell, M. F., and Maynard, L. A. 1935. The effect of retarded growth upon the length of life span and upon the ultimate body size. J. Nutr. 10: 63–79.

McCay, C. M., Maynard, L. A., Sperling, G., and Barnes, L. L. 1939. Retarded growth, life span, ultimate body size and age changes in the albino rat after feeding diets restricted in calories. J. Nutr. 18: 1–13.

Margaria, R., and Foa, P. 1939. Der Einfluss von Muskelarbeit auf den Stickstoffwechsel, die Kreatin und Saureausscheidung. (The influence of muscular work on nitrogen exchange, creatine and acid exchange.) Arbeitsphysiologie 10: 553–560.

Murlin, J. R., Edwards, L. E., Hawley, E. E., and Clark, L. C. 1946. Biological value of proteins in relation to the essential amino acids which they contain. J. Nutr. 31: 533–554.

Nocker, J. 1951. Eiweibstoffwechsel und muskelarbeit. (Protein metabolism and muscular work.) Dtsch. Z. Verdau. Stoffwechselkr. 11: 69–83.

Norgan, N. G., Ferro-Luzzi, A., and Durnin, J. V. G. A. 1974. The energy and nutrient intake and the energy expenditure of 204 New Guinean adults. Phil. Trans. R. Soc. Lond. Brit. 268: 309–348.

Périssé, J., Sizaret, F., and Francois, P. 1969. The effect of income on the structure of diet. FAO Nutr. Newsletter 7, no. 3: 1–9.

Pettenkofer, M., and Voit, C. 1866. Untersuchungen über den Stoffverbrauch des normalen Menschen. (Investigations into the nutritional consumption of normal people.) Z. Biol. 2: 459–573.

Playfair, L. 1865. On the food of man in relation to his useful work. Proc. R. Instit. 4: 431–433.

Stucke, K., Fischer, V., Feldmeier, H., and Henn, L. 1972. Fordening des Trainingsniveaus durch hochkonzentrierte Eiweisszufuhr. (Promotion of training levels by addition of highly concentrated protein.) Munch. Med. Wochensch. 114: 496–503.

Thomas, K. 1910. Uber das physiologische Stickstoffminimum. (On the physiological minimum of Nitrogen.) Arch. Physiol. Suppl.: 249–285.

Voit, C. 1881. Physiologie des allgemeinen Stoffwechsels und der Ernährung. (Physiology of general metabolism and nutrition.) In L. Hermann (ed.), Handbuch der Physiologie, Vol. VI. Vogel, Leipzig.

Von Liebig, J. 1842. In J. Owne (ed.), Animal Chemistry. Cambridge.

Wilson, H. E. C. 1932. The influence of muscular work on protein metabolism. J. Physiol. 75: 67−80.

Yamaji, R. 1951a. J. Physiol. Soc. Japan 13: 476.

Yamaji, R. 1951b. J. Physiol. Soc. Japan, 13: 483.

Yoshimura, H. 1970. Anemia during physical training (sports anemia). Nutr. Rev. 28: 251−253.

Zuntz, N. 1911. Umsatz der Nahrstoffe. (Conversion of Nutrients.) Oppenheimer's Hand. Biochem. 4: 826−881.

Body Composition and Lipid Metabolism in Relation to Nutrition and Exercise

J. Pařízková

Absolute and relative amounts of fat deposits and lean body mass ("body composition") reflect, inter alia, the nutritional status of the organism under conditions of a different balance between energy intake and output, which depends mainly on nutrition and physical activity. Adaptation to various degrees of work load modifies significantly the caloric intake, together with a number of metabolic characteristics, including lipid metabolism, which finally is manifested in changes of depot fat and lean body mass ratios. These variations are closely related to the performance capacity of the organism (Pařízková, 1963, 1973, 1977).

On the other hand, it is not necessary to stress that adequate nutrition from the beginning of life is indispensable for the desirable development of the body and its functional capacity. Chronic malnutrition in very early periods of life prevents the development of the full potentialities of the organism from morphological, mental, functional, and metabolical points of view—even when later adequate nutrition is ensured (FAO, 1962; Widdowson and McCance, 1963; Fomon, 1974; Winick, Brasel, and Rosso, 1974). This is reflected also in the aerobic, glycolytic, etc. capacity of individual muscles (Raju, 1974). However, an excessive caloric intake during the earliest period of life, resulting, e.g., in a possible disposition for developing excess fat in later life, could mean a handicap from the functional point of view, especially when considering the capacity for dynamic, aerobic exercise. The above-mentioned nutritional manipulations can cause apparent morphological and functional changes even when they are not extreme; these factors have not yet been satisfactorily studied in greater detail and from a more comprehensive aspect.

MODIFICATIONS OF CALORIC INTAKE, BODY COMPOSITION, AND LIPID METABOLISM RELATED TO EXERCISE OR HYPOKINESIA DURING POSTNATAL LIFE OF RATS

Body weight and fat proportions were always lowest in exercising animals (run daily on a motor-driven treadmill since the 18th day of life for 2–3 hr per day, with a speed up to 18 m/min,—i.e., medium or mild exercise of an aerobic character) with the highest caloric intake (Table 1). Highest weight and fat together with the lowest caloric intake were found in hypokinetic animals (housed in spaces $8 \times 12 \times 20$ cm since weaning). These differences were most apparent after the end of exponential growth, i.e., approximately at 100–120 days of age. Additional exercise can manifest its impact in adult life relatively more markedly (Pařízková 1968a; 1977) when the level of spontaneous physical activity is already declining (Smith and Dugal, 1965). Moreover, a higher level of metabolic activity was found in the adipose tissue in exercised animals (Pařízková and Staňková, 1964); experiments with injected [^{14}C] palmitate showed a lower inflow rate of fatty acids into the adipose tissue of the exercised animals, even when measured 24 hr after the last work load on the treadmill. On the other hand, the inflow rate of [^{14}C] palmitate into the heart and soleus muscle under the same conditions was significantly higher in the exercised animals (Pařízková and Poledne, 1974), indicating a higher utilization of lipid metabolites after adaptation to aerobic exercise. This was also proved by a higher level of lipoprotein lipase activity in the soleus and heart muscles (Pařízková and Koutecký, 1968), as well as an increased proportion of [^{14}C] O_2 in the expired air during the infusion of [^{14}C] palmitate into the femoral vein during pentobarbital anesthesia. Hypokinesia mostly caused changes of an opposite character (Poledne and Pařízková, 1975). The characteristically modified proportion of fat deposits resulted from a number of complex metabolic changes in the organism induced by long-term adaptation to a changed physical activity regimen—i.e., both by increased caloric intake and output in the exercised animals, or their reduced levels in the hypokinetic animals (Pařízková, 1977). Some of the mentioned contrasts are similar to differences between young and old animals. An appropriate level of physical activity seems therefore to play an important role in the fat metabolism (Issekutz et al., 1965, Paul, 1975) and in the regulation of body composition (Pařízková, 1963, 1977; Behnke and Wilmore, 1974). As follows from the above-mentioned experiments, lack of physical activity cannot be compensated for by a reduced caloric intake (Pařízková, 1977).

Mentioned changes in body composition, caloric intake, and lipid metabolism were manifested after adaptation to sufficiently intensive dynamic exercise of an aerobic character. When following these

Table 1a. Mean values of body composition, caloric intake, outflow rate of plasma-free fatty acids, and their inflow rate into the adipose tissue, soleus muscle, and heart in male rats[a]

Factors		90-day-old group			150-day-old group		
		Exercised	Control	Hypokinetic	Exercised	Control	Hypokinetic
N		11	13	12	12	12	12
Weight (g)	$\bar{x}$	342.2	380.7	345.1	430.3	445.3	487.5
	SD	11.8	25.1	26.9	27.3	44.3	43.8
Fat (%)	$\bar{x}$	5.9	12.7	12.1	9.3	16.2	18.4
	SD	1.3	3.0	2.9	2.5	2.8	3.0
Plasma volume (ml)	$\bar{x}$	13.15	12.00	12.00	15.80	13.62	14.90
	SD	1.09	1.12	0.81	1.25	1.20	1.05
Plasma FFA (μmole/ml)	$\bar{x}$	0.49	0.51	0.29	0.87	0.92	0.60
	SD	0.23	0.13	0.07	0.15	0.20	0.17
FFA pool (μmole)	$\bar{x}$	6.62	6.12	3.36	13.75	12.53	8.94
	SD	1.43	1.22	0.85	1.14	2.82	1.43
Outflow rate (μmole/min) R^a	$\bar{x}$	8.27	7.65	4.40	14.47	13.19	9.41
	SD						
Inflow rate adipose tissue (mmole/min/g tissue)	$\bar{x}$	1.96	4.15	1.86	3.11	6.46	3.86
	SD	0.55	0.82	0.33	0.62	0.85	0.41

[a] Pařízková and Poledne (1974); Poledne and Pařízková (1975); Pařízková (1977a, in press).

Table 1b.   Caloric intake of male rats

Age (days)	Group		Caloric intake (g Larsen diet/100 g body weight/liters/day) (days)				
			55−65	66−76	77−87	85−105	130−150
90	Exercised	x̄	9.9	9.7	8.0		
		SD	0.8	0.8	1.0		
	Control	x̄	9.9	9.0	8.0		
		SD	0.7	0.9	1.3		
	Hypokinetic	x̄	9.2	7.5	7.3		
		SD	1.0	0.8	1.2		
150	Exercised	x̄				7.9	6.1
		SD				1.2	0.7
	Control	x̄				7.3	4.7
		SD				0.5	0.5
	Hypokinetic	x̄				6.6	4.8
		SD				0.8	0.4

changes after static exercise (i.e., in the experimental animals hanging on vertical ladders for 3−4 hr per day), no significant changes were found (Pařízková, 1977).

BODY FAT RELATED TO DIET AND TRAINING IN ATHLETES

Changes of a similar character were found also in human subjects during periods of different intensity of training: e.g., the deposits of fat in gymnasts decreased in spite of an increased caloric intake when training was intensive, but increased after interruption of training, even when the caloric intake was markedly reduced (Pařízková and Poupa, 1963). Increased intensity of exercise caused the reduction of fat deposits in human subjects in spite of the same relative weight of compared trained and untrained subjects (Pařízková, 1963). This applied to all age categories: preschool (Pařízková et al., 1974; Pařízková and Berdychová, 1976), adolescence (Pařízková, 1968a,b, 1972a), and adult and advanced age (Pařízková and Eiselt, 1966, Pařízková, 1977).

Most marked changes were found in adult top athletes where the intensity of training was highest. In this case there was also a differentiation of dynamic and static sport disciplines: the lowest relative weight and depot fat ratio was found, e.g., in long distance runners (Pařízková, 1972b), who achieved the highest levels of aerobic capacity. Members of static sports disciplines, e.g., weight lifters and wrestlers, had not only an increased body weight but, especially in higher weight categories, the values of fat ratio were above levels usually considered borderline for obesity. The aerobic capacity was

Table 2. Mean values of height, weight, body composition, and aerobic capacity in top athletes of dynamic and static sport disciplines[a]

Characteristic	Runners (N = 10)		Weight lifters (N = 14)	
	x̄	SD	x̄	SD
Age (years)	22.5	5.0	24.9	3.4
Height (cm)	177.3	5.0	166.3	7.8
Weight (kg)	64.5	5.0	77.1	14.9
Lean body mass (%)	93.7	1.8	90.1	5.1
Fat (kg)	4.1	1.4	8.1	5.7
Max O_2 (liters/min)	4.13	0.27	3.29	0.33
Max O_2 (kg weight)	64.1	2.3	43.6	5.9
Max O_2 (kg lean body mass)	68.4	2.5	48.4	5.8
Max O_2 pulse	22.0	1.3	17.3	1.9

[a] Šprynarová and Pařízková (1971).

low in this case (Šprynarová and Pařízková, 1971) (Table 2). Caloric intake related to body weight was increased, compared to the normal sedentary population, in both cases. Highest weight and fatness was found in Sumo wrestlers (Suzuki et al., 1961), who had a very high caloric intake and mainly static training. In these athletes elevated insulin levels and prediabetic changes after glucose tolerance test appeared; the hyperresponse of insulin decreased significantly with weight reduction (Kuzuya, Akanuma, and Kosaka, 1975). As is apparent, only specified types of work load can influence in a positive way the aerobic capacity, lipid metabolism, and body fatness (Pařízková, 1977); therefore, "jogging" or similar exercise is recommended as a preventive measure against metabolic and cardiovascular diseases. Differing kinds of fitness and performance capacities in individual disciplines of top sports must be specified; they do not always imply the best overall general physical fitness and optimal health status desirable for the normal population with regard to health prognosis (Pařízková, 1977).

NUTRITION AND OTHER FACTORS INFLUENCING PHYSICAL ACTIVITY, MOTOR DEVELOPMENT, AND FATNESS

Especially in top sports, *genetic and constitutional predispositions* are assumed to play a very important role in the achievement of highest level of performance. In the normal population, apparent differences in the level of spontaneous physical activity and motor skill, etc. can also be found that mostly seem to be of an inborn character. The range of spontaneous physical activity per unit of time varies markedly, as measured both in experimental animals and human subjects, even when other characteristics (age, sex, living conditions, etc.) are nearly identical; however, in one individual it is fairly stable (Slonin and Smirnov, 1972). Monozygotic twins are more similar than dizygotic twins in the total volume of physical activity (Ledovskaya, 1972), as well as in the structure of movements during special tasks (Sklad, 1972).

A wide range of variability in caloric intake in homogeneous population groups was described long ago (Widdowson, 1962). There is an interesting empirical observation that in groups of specialized top athletes—e.g., in racing cyclists, who belong to one of the most demanding sport disciplines—the caloric intake of competitors who engage in identical training programs could differ markedly (even by 100% in individual cases, which cannot be explained by different weight, etc.), indicating that different mechanisms cause a varying energy expenditure for the same activity. The background of these differences, as well as variations in physical activity levels or a wide range of caloric intake under apparently similar conditions, are not yet fully elucidated. Different metabolic patterns in individual subjects with a different functional capacity, body composition, and physique deserve further experimental study.

Except for genetic factors, the *influence of various factors starting with nutrition and activity during the earliest periods of ontogeny, both pre- and postnatal,* ought to be considered. As mentioned above, different nutrition in early stages of growth (i.e., weaning in nests with a different number of pups) influences the size and cellularity of the epididymal fat pads in later life (Knittle and Hirsch, 1968). Oscai et al. (1974) described a significant decrease in epididymal fat pad size and cellularity in male rats of adult age (64 weeks) that swam daily, starting on the 5th day of life and continuing until the age of 28 weeks. Both nutrition and exercise at the beginning of life changed the later development of the adipose tissue in the organism. For that reason, the interrelationships between nutrition and spontaneous physical activity after similar early manipulations in nutrition have also been studied.

Experimental animals (male rats, Wistar strain) were weaned in nests of up to six pups, or above 12 pups—i.e., those who had more or less mother's milk for their nutrition in this early period of life were weaned. After weaning (30th day of life), they were kept under the same experimental conditions: five animals per cage and on the same diet ad libitum. In the first series of experiments the level of spontaneous physical activity was measured in the rotation cages together with the caloric intake. Body weight was lower in the animals from bigger nests, but only until the 62nd day of life (See Table 3). The spontaneous

Table 3. Mean values of body weight, distance covered spontaneously in rotation cages, and caloric intake in male rats weaned from nests by more than 12 or less than 6 pups

Number of pups per litter		56–62 days		Caloric intake (g/100 g weight/day)	69–74 days		Caloric intake (g/100 g weight/day)	75–79 days		Caloric intake (g/100 g weight(day))
		Weight (g)	m/day		Weight (g)	m/day		Weight	m/day	
>12	x̄	248	3,372	11.9	324	6,088	8.7	350	7,390	10.7
	SD	22	1,813	1.0	30	1,933	0.6	34	956	0.2
<6	x̄	278	2,261	10.6	306	2,855	9.2	341	4,032	11.1
	SD	33	500	0.9	36	559	0.3	36	493	0.8

physical activity tended to be higher since the beginning measurements in the animals from bigger nests, and this difference was significant in the period from the 69–79th day of life; the mean distance in meters covered per day was nearly twice as long in the animals from bigger nests. Caloric intake related to body weight was mostly similar in both experimental groups until the age of 79 days and did not differ from the caloric intake of animals measured previously, weaned eight per one nest (Table 3).

The results concerning changes in spontaneous physical activity as a result of early nutrition were verified in another, longer series of experiments that also included females. In males from bigger nests, the level of spontaneous physical activity increased permanently, but in the males from smaller nests it increased only up to the 57th day of life (i.e., puberty—see Figure 1). On the other hand, the level of spontaneous physical activity in females was higher in those from bigger nests only at the age of 50–57 days of life. Further measurements revealed that the females from smaller nests achieved similar high values as those from bigger nests, and finally there were no differences between both groups of females and the group of males from bigger nests (Figure 1).

Figure 2 shows caloric intake and weight development. Body weight of males from bigger nests was significantly smaller; in females

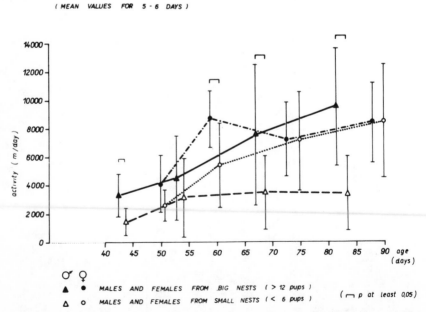

Figure 1. Development of spontaneous physical activity in male and female rats with different nutrition during weaning period.

there were no differences. Caloric intake related to body weight did not differ during the acceleration period of growth; at the end of the measurements the males from bigger nests with more intense physical activity also had a higher caloric intake, but only in the period from 80–84 days of life. In females no differences were observed (Pařízková, in press).

The absolute weights of individual organs (heart, soleus muscle, adrenals) did not differ. When related to total body weight they tended to be higher in males from bigger nests. Epididymal fat pads were significantly lighter in males from bigger nests, and also the percentage of total body fat was lower (10.3%) than in males from smaller nests with lower activity (11.1%), in spite of a higher caloric intake during the last period of the experiment (Figure 2) (Pařízková, in press).

Selected indicators of the lipid metabolism measured in total carcass, liver, and small intestine varied in the mentioned groups. When following the total activity of cholesterol (measured after the administration of [^{14}C] acetate, expressed as percentage of total activity injected), it was higher in the carcass of males from smaller nests. Total lipids (g/100 ml), lipogenesis, and the synthesis of fatty acids in the small intestine were significantly reduced in the animals of both sexes

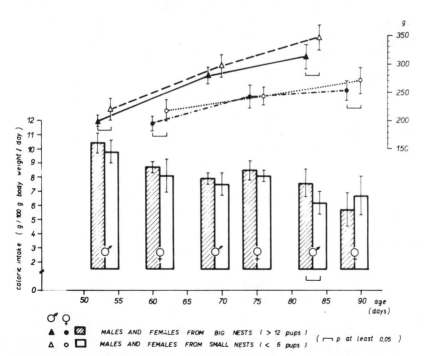

Figure 2. Development of body weight and caloric intake in male and female rats with different nutrition during weaning period.

from small nests. The concentration of fatty acids in the liver was significantly lower in both males and females from smaller nests. There were some differences between sexes with regard to their reaction to changed early nutrition (Pařízková and Petrásek, in press b). Cholesterolemia did not differ.

Mentioned results confirm a marked impact of the nutrition during very early periods of life, which extend also to the later motor development and spontaneous level of physical activity, caloric intake, and selected parameters of lipid metabolism. Even when the differences in the nutrition during weaning were not so great as in experiments of other authors, the later development of the animals differed in many ways. The impact of changed nutrition in early life was not the same in both sexes, at least during the period of life observed. In animals similarly differentiated according to early nutrition, Macho, Štrbák, and Hromadová, (1973) found increased activity of the thyroid gland. Smart (1974) showed that rats from mothers who were undernourished during much of the pregnancy and throughout lactation were more active than controls in familiar, nonstressful situations. Sadile, Lát, and Cioffi (1977) also proved increased excitability of the central nervous system after puberty in rats weaned in larger nests compared to those from smaller nests, which can be related to the development of spontaneous physical activity, and both directly and indirectly to the changes of caloric intake and lipid metabolism. Mechanisms underlying the *different programming of future motor activity as a result of early nutrition,* as well as the sexual differences in the reaction to it, cannot be explained completely from the author's data, or from other available data in the literature. These problems deserve further experimental explanation from the point of view of individual differentiation in motor activity, physique and body composition, caloric intake, and lipid metabolism.

IMPACT OF EXERCISE DURING
PRENATAL ONTOGENY ON FUTURE DEVELOPMENT

Nutritional status and caloric intake of the mother during pregnancy can profoundly change future morphological, metabolical, or mental development of the offspring (Winick, Brasel, and Rosso, 1974). With regard to exercise, Arshavsky (1967) showed that newborns of hare mothers that swam daily during the last third of pregnancy were born with larger hearts.

Offspring of rat mothers that exercised for 1 hr daily on a treadmill (speed 14–15 m/min), starting with the 2nd or 3rd day after mating, were therefore studied. Total body weights at birth and during as well as at the end of experiment did not differ. Fifty- and 100-day-old male offspring were studied from the point of view of the microstructure of the heart muscle, which has an important relationship to the functional capacity of the cardiovascular system. Figure 3 shows that the weights of the hearts in the offspring of exercised mothers were significantly heavier, the number of fibers and capillaries per sq mm was higher, the capillary:fiber ratio was higher, and the diffusion distance was smaller (Pařízková, 1975, 1977). These comparisons show better functional disposition of the heart muscle in the offspring of mothers that exercised regularly during pregnancy. This can have a positive impact on the performance capacity of the organism later in life.

The mechanisms of these changes resulting from regular exercise during pregnancy are not fully explained. As is generally known, regular work loads change some metabolic parameters in the blood (level of glucose, pyruvate, lactate, free fatty acids, etc.; increased release of catecholamines, etc.), change hemodynamics in the organism (possible increase of placental blood flow per unit of time), and so forth. Because of changes in her interior milieu, the fetus of the exercised mother obviously gets more metabolic, hemodynamic, hormonal, etc. stimuli, which might change the programming of its postnatal life. This can be manifested not only in the body size, nutritional status, and so forth, but also in functional capacity of the organism.

The impact of exercise during pregnancy can be manifested in the lipid metabolism of the offspring. When selected parameters were examined (e.g., in the liver), a significant change was found, especially

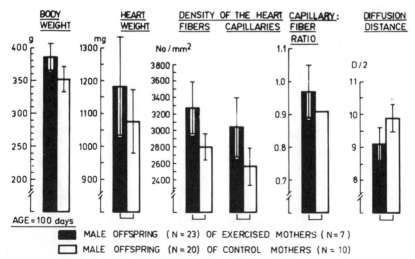

Figure 3. Comparison of male offspring of rat mothers exercised during pregnancy to control mothers.

Table 4. Mean values of body weight and the concentration of total lipids and fatty acids in the liver of the offspring of rat mothers exercised during pregnancy (E) and of control mothers (C)[a]

Sex and group	Body Weight (g) at 35 days		Total lipids (g/100 ml) at 35 days		Fatty acids (g/100 ml) at 35 days		Body weight (g) at 90 days		Total lipids (g/100 ml) at 90 days		Fatty acids (g/100 ml) at 90 days	
	$\bar{x}$	SD	$\bar{x}$	SD	$\bar{x}$	SD	$\bar{x}$	SD	$\bar{x}$	SD	$\bar{x}$	SD
Female (C)	99	3.5	4.98	0.17	2.89	0.54	245	12.3	5.26	0.25	3.80	0.15
Female (E)	104	3.6	5.70	0.13	3.54	0.11	240	9.1	5.93	0.21	4.27	0.23
Male (C)	92	6.3	5.37	0.25	3.56	0.21	366	11.4	5.23	0.22	3.90	0.20
Male (E)	101	3.1	4.99	0.16	3.51	0.15	335	17.2	5.22	0.11	3.67	0.13

[a] Pařízková and Petrásek (in press).

in female offspring of mothers exercised during pregnancy, similar to the type described above. The concentration of total lipids and fatty acids (assessed gravimetrically) in the liver was significantly increased in female offspring of exercised mothers, together with their decreased synthesis (Table 4). In males, such changes were either not apparent or were of reverse character. Blood levels of free fatty acids were significantly higher in both female and male offspring of exercised rat mothers (Pařízková and Petrásek, in press; Pařízková et al., in press a). There were also changes in the lipid metabolism in the small intestine as a result of the exercise by the mother (Pařízková and Petrásek, in press). The exercise of the mother during pregnancy also changed the reaction to the adaptation to exercise during postnatal ontogeny of the offspring (Pařízková and Petrásek, in press b).

CONCLUSIONS

Relationships between nutrition and physical activity regimens significantly influence the activity of lipid metabolism when modified in both a positive (increased energy input and output) or negative (reduced activity resulting mostly in decreased caloric intake) way, together with depot fat and lean, fat-free body mass ratios. However, *restricted activity cannot be compensated for by a decline in caloric intake,* and marked modifications of lipid metabolism develop simultaneously with excess deposits of fat; this was found both in laboratory animals and in human subjects. Dynamic exercise of an aerobic character seems to cause favorable changes in lipid metabolism, i.e., increasing its activity (resembling thus the state usually found in younger developmental stages), which results also in the limited deposit of fat. This does not appear after static exercise paralleled mostly by a reduced aerobic capacity of the organism. Further experimental data indicate remarkable importance of both nutrition and physical activity regime during the earliest periods of life—including prenatal ontogeny—for the further development of metabolic pattern including lipids, heart muscle, and so forth, which are all closely related to the level of functional capacity of the organism. Great individual variations existing in human subjects and many other species mostly elucidated by genetics and inborn constitutional qualities of the organism could be better explained by various manipulations during the earliest periods of life, including diet and motor activity regimens.

REFERENCES

Arshavsky, I. A. 1967. Some Aspects of Developmental Physiology. Moscow.
Behnke A. R. Jr., and Willmore, J. 1974. Evaluation and Regulation of Body Build and Composition. Prentice-Hall, Englewood Cliffs, N.J.
Fomon, S. J. 1974. Infant Nutrition. 2nd ed., W.B. Saunders Co. New York.

FAO. 1962. Basic Study, 5.

Issekutz, B., Jr., Miller, H., Paul, P., and Rodahl, K. 1965. Aerobic work capacity and plasma free fatty acid turnover. J. Appl. Physiol. 20: 293.

Knittle, J., and Hirsch, J. 1968. Effect of early nutrition on the development of epididymal fat pads: Cellularity and metabolism. J. Clin. Invest. 47: 2091.

Kuzuya, T., Akanuma, Y., and Kosaka, K. 1975. Carbohydrate metabolism in obesity . . . with special reference to the relationship of glucose intolerance and insulin hyperresponse. In H. Koishi et al. (eds.), Proc. Xth Int. Congr. Nutr., Kyoto, Aug. 3–9 , p. 262.

Ledovskaya, N. M. 1972. A study of physical activity in twin children. In A.D. Slonim and K.M. Smirnov (eds.), Physical Activity in Man and Hypokinesia, p. 30. Academy of Sciences USSR, Siberian Branch, Novosibirsk.

Macho, L., Štrbák, V., and Hromadová, A. M. 1973. Effect of early undernutrition and overnutrition on thyroid gland function in rats. Endocrinologia 62: 194.

Oscai, L. B., Babirak, S. P., Dubach, F. B., McGarr, J. A., and Spirakis, C. N. 1974. Effect of exercise on adipose tissue cellularity. Am. J. Physiol. 227: 901.

Pařízková, J. 1963. The impact of age, diet and exercise on man's body composition. Ann. N.Y Acad. Sci. 110: 661.

Pařízková, J. 1968a. Compositional growth in relation to metabolic activity. Proc. XIIth. Int. Cong. Pediatr., Mexico City I: 32.

Pařízková, J. 1968b. Longitudinal study of body composition and body build development in boys of various physical activity, from 11 to 15 years. Hum. Biol. 40: 212.

Pařízková, J. 1972a. Somatic development and body composition changes in adolescent boys differing in physical activity and fitness: A longitudinal study. Anthropologia 10: 3.

Pařízková, J. 1972b. La masse active, la graisse dépote et la constitution corporelle chez les sportifs du haut niveau. (Lean body mass, fat deposits and body composition of high level sportsmen.) Kinanthropologie 4: 95.

Pařízková, J. 1973. Body composition and exercise during growth and development. In L.G. Rarick (ed.), Physical Activity: Human Growth and Development, p. 97. Academic Press, New York.

Pařízková, J. 1974. Body composition, nutrition and exercise. Med. Sport 27: 2.

Pařízková, J. 1975. Impact of daily work load during pregnancy on the microstructure of the rat heart in male offspring. Europ. J. Appl. Physiol. 34: 1.

Pařízková, J. 1977. Body Fat and Physical Fitness. Martinus Nighoff, B.V./ Medical Division, The Hague.

Pařízková, J. Nutrition and functional capacity. Proc. Symp. Indian Nutr. Soc., Jan. 27, 1977. In press.

Pařízková, J. and Berdychová, J. 1976. The level of somatic and motor development in preschool children. Proc. Conf. Int. FIEPS—Education Physique avant la Puberté, May 27–31. Editions Scientifiques de Pologne, p. 506, Varsovie-Poznan.

Pařízková, J., Čermák, J., and Horná, J. 1974. Nutritional requirements, somatic and functional development of preschool children. G. Débry and R. Blayer (eds.), Proc. 2ème Symp. Int. Alimentation et Travail, p. 37.

Pařízková, J., and Eiselt, E. 1966. Body composition and anthropometric indicators in old age and the influence of physical exercise. Hum. Biol. 38: 351.

Pařízková, J., and Eiselt, E. 1968. Longitudinal study of changes in anthropometric indicators and body composition in old men of various physical activity. Hum. Biol. 40: 331.

Pařízková, J., and Koutecký, Z. 1968. The effect of age and different motor activity on fat content, lipoproteine-lipase activity and relative weight of internal organs, heart and skeletal muscle. Physiol. Bohemoslov. 17: 177.

Pařízková, J., and Petrásek, R. Changes in the microstructure of the heart and lipid metabolism of the offspring of rats exercised during pregnancy. Proc. Int. Conf. Nutrition, Dietetics, and Sport, June 7–9, 1976, Bordighera. Medicina dello Sporte. In press a.

Pařízková, J., and Petrásek, R. The impact of daily work load during pregnancy on lipid metabolism in the liver of the offspring. Europ. J. Appl. Physiol. In press b.

Pařízková, J., and Poledne, R. 1974. Consequences of long term hypokinesia as compared to mild exercise on lipid metabolism of the heart, skeletal muscle and adipose tissue. Europ. J. Appl. Physiol. 33: 331.

Pařízková, J., Poledne, R., and Petrásek, R. Body composition, lipid metabolism, physical activity and nutrition. Proc. Int. Congress Phys. Activity Sciences, July 11–16, 1976, Quebec City. In press.

Pařízková, J., and Poupa, O. 1963. Some metabolic consequences of adaptation to muscular work. Brit. J. Nutr. 17: 341.

Pařízková, J., and Staňková, L. 1964. Influence of physical activity on a treadmill on the metabolism of adipose tissue in rats. Brit. J. Nutr. 18: 325.

Paul, P. 1975. Effects of long lasting exercise and training on lipid metabolism. In H. Howald and J.R. Poortmans (eds.), Metabolic Adaptation to Prolonged Exercise, p. 156. Birkhäuser Verlag, Basel.

Petrásek, R., and Pařízková, J. 1975. Cholesterol formation in rat liver induced by various levels of physical activity. Physiol. Bohemoslov. 24: 462.

Poledne, R., and Pařízková, J. 1975. Long term training and net transport of plasma free fatty acids. In H. Howald and J.R. Poortmans (eds.), Metabolic Adaptation to Prolonged Exercise, p. 201. Birkhäuser Verlag, Basel.

Raju, N. V. 1974. Effect of early malnutrition on muscle function and metabolism in rats. Life Sci. 15: 949.

Sadile, A. G., Lát, J., and Cioffi, L. A. 1977. Late effects of early postnatal malnutrition on spontaneous exploratory activity in rats. Act. Nerv. Sup. 19: 135.

Sklad, M. 1972. Similarity of movements in twins. Wych. Fiz. Sport 3: 119.

Slonin, A. D., and Smirnov, K. M. 1972. Physical activity in man and hypokinesia. Acad. Sci. USSR, Siberian branch, Novosibirsk.

Smart, J. L. 1974. Activity and exploratory behavior of adult offspring of undernourished mothers. Dev. Psychobiol. 7: 315.

Smith, L. C., and Dugal, L. P. 1965. Age and spontaneous running activity in male rats. Can. J. Physiol. Pharmacol. 43: 852.

Šprynarová, Š., and Pařízková, J. 1971. Functional capacity and body composition in top weight-lifters, swimmers, runners and skiers. Int. Ztschr. Angew. Physiol. 29: 185.

Suzuki, S., Kuga, T., Oshima, S., et al. 1961. Studies of the nutrition of the Sportsman (report 2). Morphological measurement of sumo-wrestlers. Japan J. Nutr. 19: 191.

Widdowson, W. 1962. Nutritional individuality. Proc. Nutr. Soc. 21: 121.

Widdowson, W., and McCance, R. A. 1963. The effect of finite periods of undernutrition at different ages on the composition and subsequent development of the rat. Proc. R. Soc. Brit. 158: 329.

Winick, M., Brasel, J. A., and Rosso, P. 1974. Nutrition and cell growth. In M. Winick and J. Wiley (eds.), Nutrition and Development, p. 49. John Wiley and Sons, New York.

Fluid, Electrolyte, and Energy Losses and Their Replenishment in Prolonged Exercise

B. Saltin

An individual's physical performance capacity is primarily restricted by the ability of the ventilation and circulation to transport, and the capacity of the muscle tissue to utilize oxygen. This applies when large muscle groups are activated continuously for more than a few minutes. A number of secondary factors influence the magnitude of performance or the duration of the exercise period when prolonged exercise is performed. Two of these factors are increasing dehydration, including electrolyte losses because of sweating, and the shortage of suitable substrate for the energy metabolism of muscles. This chapter examines certain aspects of these two problems.

HEAT BALANCE

Temperature in Various Body Tissues During Prolonged Exercise

During exercise the body's core temperature (CNS, thorax, abdominal cavity) is at a higher level. This applies to a wide range of work loads and varying ambient temperatures. In his notable experiments, Nielsen (1938) demonstrated that rectal temperature after about 30 min of exercise had adjusted to the new level, which was then maintained until the completion of exercise, returning to the normal rest level within a half hour. The steady-state temperature during exercise is related to exercise intensity, and it is the relative load that determines

The original results reported in this review have been supported by grants from the Danish Sport Federation.

core temperature (Saltin and Hermansen, 1966). However, there are certain situations—e.g., swimming, light work without clothing in very cold weather, and heavy work in very warm surroundings—in which the regulatory mechanisms are incapable of maintaining heat balance.

The temperatures in the skin and the muscle are also of interest from the point of view of heat regulation (Saltin, Gagge, and Stolwijk, 1968, 1970). Muscle temperature at rest is usually less than core temperature, but rises very quickly when muscles are put to work. With an ambient temperature of 20°C, the temperature gradient between the warmest part of the muscle and arterial blood or core temperature is about 0.6°C. Skin temperature is not affected by work intensity, but ambient temperature has a direct influence. This is seen in Figure 1, which shows mean skin temperature with three different work levels and ambient temperatures. Irrespective of work load, skin temperature is approximately 28, 30.5, and 33°C when ambient temperature is 10, 20, and 30°C, respectively (Stolwijk, Saltin, and Gagge, 1968).

The Magnitude of Sweating During Work

There is heat exchange with the surroundings (Figure 2) so that a constant body temperature may be maintained at different levels of energy metabolism. When heat exchange via convection, radiation,

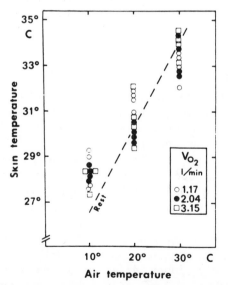

Figure 1. Mean skin temperature at rest and at three metabolic rates (bicycle exercise) in three environments (relative humidity < 40%). The symbols denote different subjects and metabolic rates (From Stolwijk, Saltin, and Gagge, 1968).

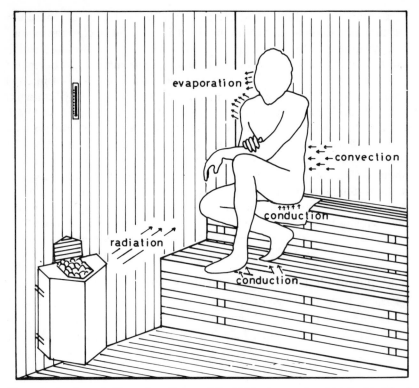

Figure 2. A schematic illustration of some of the different means by which heat is gained or dissipated from the body.

conduction, and respiratory channels (insensible water loss) are insufficient, water also evaporates from the skin (sweat). In windless conditions, about 7 kcal disappear per hr and m^2 of body area (8 w/m^2 through radiation and convection per degree of temperature gradient between skin and surroundings) (Nishi and Gagge, 1970). In steady-state conditions, remaining heat (heat stored in the body [S] at the beginning of work may be generally ignored) is disposed of through sweating, the magnitude of which can be calculated from the equation $M^\pm S^\pm (R+C)$, in which M stands for heat production through energy metabolism, R+C for radiation and convection, and E for the heat consumed in the evaporation of water. This evaporation is mainly from the skin. When air temperature exceeds 32°C, the disposal of water via respiratory channels is limited (Barr et al., 1968).

Even with very heavy loads in warm surroundings, sweating does not start until after 1/2−3 min of work have been performed; it then displays a linear increase until leveling off after 10−15 min of work

(Saltin, Gagge, and Stolwijk, 1968). The body's core temperature does not change in step with sweating when work is begun, but skin and muscle temperature, taken together, co-vary with sweating ($r = 0.88$). In steady-state conditions, the correlation coefficient between skin, muscle, and core temperature and sweating is 0.96 (Saltin, Gagge, and Stolwijk, 1968, 1970). Thus, good co-variation between temperature in different tissues and the magnitude of sweating can be demonstrated. However, it is not certain that these temperatures alone are active in the regulation of sweating. The existence of a factor unrelated to a tissue temperature in the body but related to, for example, the absolute magnitude of energy output may be required to provide a complete explanation of perspiration regulation during exercise (Snellen, 1966). Even if regulation of the magnitude of sweating cannot be explained completely, available studies show that there is very accurate control, and almost identical levels of sweating intensity are noted if equally well acclimatized persons work with the same absolute load in the same surroundings (Saltin and Hermansen, 1966).

A theoretical calculation of fluid losses through sweating is relatively easy to make with the aid of the above equation, at least with cycling and running, in which the degree of mechanical efficiency is known. It is around 20% in these forms of exercise, which means that the remaining 80% of energy metabolism is converted into heat. Certain calculated and measured values for fluid losses during exercise are shown in Table 1 with different ambient temperatures. The values indicate that a fluid loss of 1−2 liters/hr is quite common at around 20°C. The observed values exceeded the estimated values because part of the

Table 1. Loss of Fluid[a]

Ambient temperature °C (no wind)	Low speed calculated (liters/hr)	High speed calculated (liters/hr)	High speed observed (liters/hr)[b]
−5°	0.3	1.1	1.1 0.6 − 1.4
+10°	0.6	1.5	1.6 1.2 − 1.5
+20°	0.9	1.8	2.0 1.6 − 2.4
+30°	1.1	2.1	2.4 2.0 − 2.8

[a] The calculated values given in the table are based on subjects with a weight of 70 kg, working with 80% of their maximal oxygen uptake; the trained subjects have maximal oxygen uptake of 5.0 liters/min, and the untrained have 3.0 liters/min uptake. It is further assumed that the clothing is adjusted to the ambient temperature.

[b] The observed values are taken from unpublished investigations in different sports.

sweat produced did not evaporate from the skin, but fell to the ground in drops or remained in clothing.

Calculations were made for windless conditions, and this causes a certain amount of error (e.g., in cycling), but the error is undoubtedly very small in other forms of exercise, or at low ambient temperatures, when clothing counteracts any major increase in heat losses through convection. However, large amounts of heat can still be given off through convection. Ten to 15 W/m^2 per degree of temperature gradient are lost when walking on a treadmill at a speed of 5 to 10 km/hr, respectively (Nishi and Gagge, 1970). Heat losses through convection are especially great from arms and legs.

ELECTROLYTE LOSSES

The exact content of sodium, chloride, potassium, and other ions in sweat cannot be given. This is partly a function of the difficulties encountered when sampling sweat, and being sure that the obtained samples truly represent all parts of the body throughout the exercise. The problem has been dealt with by many researchers, and good critical reviews are available (Robinson and Robinson, 1954; Kuno, 1956; Vellar, 1969). Table 2 furnishes some values for ion losses obtained in sampled sweat. The data are taken from Vellar's work (1969), in which he had rather high sweat intensities and partly heat-acclimatized subjects, who had normal water and electrolyte stores at the start of the experiment. Thus, the loss of 2 mM/liter of sodium and 2 mM/liter of chloride can be expected to be substantially lower in the heat-acclimatized persons, and may be twice as high in completely unacclimatized subjects when sweating profusely.

The Effect of Dehydration on the Body's Fluid Volume

Water and electrolytes for production of sweat by sweat glands come primarily from extracellular sources. These sources comprise plasma water and interstitial tissue water. There is a rapid exchange of water between plasma water and extravascular sources. Even if total body water declines in work, it would seem that the level of plasma water is retained to the very last (Koszlowski and Saltin, 1964; Saltin and Stenberg, 1965; Ekelund, 1967), which means, in turn, that water losses in absolute figures are primarily made up from intracellular water.

The result is intracellular dehydration with impaired cellular metabolism. Because perspiration is hypotonic, extracellular water tends to become hypertonic, a circumstance that contributes to intracellular dehydration. On the other hand, the osmolality in the exer-

Table 2.   Comparisons between the concentrations of various constituents in arm-bag sweat with the corresponding concentrations in whole body sweat[a]

Variable		Arm-bag sweat (mean ± SE)	Whole body sweat (mean ± SE)
Cl	(mEq/liter)	46.5 ± 7.0 (5)	50.0 ± 2.4 (27)
Na	(mEq/liter)	54.5 ± 8.4 (5)	59.1 ± 4.4 (10)
K	(mEq/liter)	6.0 ± 0.1 (5)	4.6 ± 0.2 (10)
Ca	(mEq/liter)	1.10 ± 0.34 (5)	0.33 ± 0.02 (27)
Mg	(mEq/liter)	0.22 ± 0.05 (5)	0.13 ± 0.02 (27)
Fe	(μg/100 ml)	38.1 ± 6.0 (5)	29.8 ± 1.8 (23)
Zn	(μg/100 ml)	35.3 ± 13.7 (5)	9.2 ± 1.5 (5)
Cu	(μg/100 ml)	214 ± 50 (5)	190 ± 47 (5)
N	(mg/100 ml)	39.9 ± 2.2	24.2 ± 1.3

[a] The numbers in parentheses indicate number of subjects. For each subject the values are based on 1–6 determinations (Vellar, 1969).

cising muscle cell may be enhanced, which partly counteracts the flux of the water from the cell (Lundvall et al., 1972).

The Effect of Dehydration on Work Ability

Several studies have shown that a reduction in body water causes a pronounced impairment of work ability with physical labor of long duration. Incompletely compensated water losses also lead to increases in body temperature and pulse rate that are greater than normal (Adolph, 1947; Saltin, 1964). This occurs when there is a fluid loss corresponding to 1% of body weight. If a loss should amount to 4–5% of body weight, the capacity for very hard, muscular work must be expected to decline by 20–30%. The risk of circulatory collapse should be very great with work in a warm environment when dehydration amounts to 10% of body weight (Adolph, 1947).

The decline in work ability with dehydration cannot be accommodated through heat acclimatization, which leads to increased sweating with a lower salt content in the sweat (Adolph, 1947). However, certain results suggest that trained persons more easily tolerate dehydration in exercise than untrained persons (Buskirk, Iampietro, and Bass, 1958; Greenleaf, 1966; Bonnesen and Rasmussen, 1976). The need for adequate water intake during exercise has, thus, been well-documented. Unfortunately, man is not able to use thirst alone to ingest the same amount of water that is lost through heavy sweating. This is particularly true during work. Only about 50% of the amount required is, in fact, taken (Adolph, 1947; Greenleaf, 1966). This has been designated as voluntary dehydration during work. It is therefore necessary to administer water beyond subjective needs during work to prevent dehydration. Forced drinking is recommended before and during work efforts of long duration. Overhydration has never been described in persons with normal renal function, nor has it been proved that increased water intake during exercise leads to a pronounced increase in sweating beyond requirements.

FUEL STORAGE AND UTILIZATION

Guided by determination of the respiratory exchange ratio (R) and its change with increasing work loads, it has long been known that both lipids and carbohydrates are utilized as substrates in muscular work (see Rosell and Saltin, 1973). Of these two sources of energy, the relative role of carbohydrates increases with higher levels of work intensity and probably reaches 100% with brief, maximum effort. This has been verified in a number of studies through direct determination of the glycogen concentration in the working musculature (Hermansen, Hultman, and Saltin, 1967; Saltin and Hermansen, 1967; Saltin and Karlsson, 1971). It was then shown that muscle glycogen was the most important substrate source for muscle with very hard work.

If glycogen supply is exhausted during work in progress, test subjects are unable to continue because of exhaustion. Any continuation of exercise requires a considerable reduction in exercise intensity. It was also shown that previously established improvements in performance following a period with extreme carbohydrate diet (Bergström et al., 1967) could be explained by the fact that glycogen concentration in muscle is elevated above the normal. The total amount of glycogen in the muscle may vary between 300 g (mixed diet) to 600–900 g (dietary manipulation, see below).

Blood and Liver

Eight to 10 g of glucose is available in the blood and in interstitial fluid. However, the main extramuscular carbohydrate stores, in addition to those built into different membranes and cell structures and therefore not immediately available for energy metabolism, are found in the liver. In different animals there are wide variations in the normal glycogen content of the liver, which may be attributable in part to species differences, but other factors—including diet and the degree of physical activity—also affect liver glycogen content. In man, after a mixed diet and no exercise during the preceding 24 hr, the liver glycogen content seems to vary between 40 and 50 g/kg (Hultman and Nilsson, 1971). With a liver weight of 1.4−1.8 kg, the total amount of glycogen stored in the liver would then be 55−90 g. One day of starvation or food intake without carbohydrates is sufficient to produce almost complete depletion of liver glycogen stores. By contrast, a carbohydrate-enriched diet for 24 hr may double the normal glycogen content (Hultman and Nilsson, 1971).

Another physiologically interesting way to estimate the magnitude of available hepatic carbohydrates is to determine the release of glucose from the splanchnic area during exercise. Here glucose may be derived from glycogenolysis in the liver as well as from gluconeogenesis. Results from several studies (Rowell, Masoro, and Spencer, 1965; Rowell et al., 1966; Hultman, 1967; Rowell, 1971) show that there is gradual enhancement of hepatic glucose release with time during exercise. Moreover, the greater the relative work load, the greater the production of glucose. During the first hour of a prolonged exercise period, 15−25 g of glucose can be supplied by the liver; a maximum rate of 30−35 g in a 1-hr period has been reported (Hultman, 1967; Wahren et al., 1971). These values are in very good agreement with the 24 g/hr reported by Hultman and Nilsson (1971). They based their calculations of liver glucose production on direct determinations of liver glycogen content after 1 hr of exercise. Rowell (1971) estimated that at the most, one-third of the glucose produced during exercise comes from gluconeogenesis. The main precursors in glucose synthesis are lactate, pyruvate, and glycerol, all of which are taken up by the liver during exercise.

Recent data in human volunteers indicate that alanine is released in significant amounts from skeletal muscle (Felig et al., 1970). This is interesting because alanine is extracted from the blood by the liver and is the principal gluconeogenic amino acid (Malette, Exton, and Park, 1969). During exercise on a bicycle ergometer, which resulted in a three- to ninefold increase in oxygen consumption, Felig and Wahren (1971a, 1971b) observed that alanine was the only amino acid released in significant amounts from the leg. The arterial concentration of alanine also rose. They suggested that alanine may be synthesized from pyruvate by transamination. The carbon skeleton of alanine may be derived from the breakdown of glucose in the working skeletal muscle. Alanine may therefore be of importance as a substrate for hepatic glucose production and, according to Felig and Wahren, may cover up to 10% of total hepatic release of glucose. The quantitative role of the alanine-glucose cycle during exercise may be modest. However, in starvation or with a noncarbohydrate diet for an extended period of time, the conversion of alanine to glucose in the liver may be an important factor in keeping blood glucose at a physiological level.

NORMAL DIETARY INTAKE OF
CARBOHYDRATES, LIPIDS, AND PROTEINS

In the Scandinavian countries, dietary habits vary within a narrow range. The intake of different nutrients is also similar at a given total energy intake. Detailed reports on this matter are available (Blix, 1965; Wretlind, 1968). Some results on different groups of athletes are added here (Saltin and Karlsson, 1972). Scandinavians have a high total energy intake, with a mean value of above 3,500 kcal/24 hr (Figure 3). As in the general population, the variation between the groups in the intake of protein, lipids, and carbohydrates is small, with mean values of 12% (11−14), 40% (38−43), and 48% (41−51). This means that they

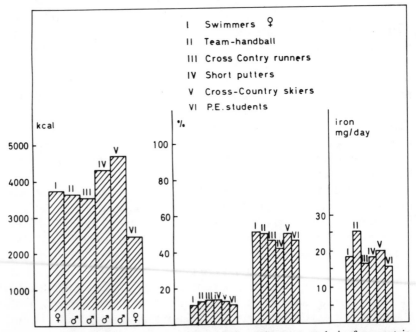

Figure 3. Mean values for total caloric intake (left panel), percent calories from protein (middle panel, left) and from carbohydrates (middle panel, right), and iron intake (right panel) for six different groups of subjects undertaking regular exercise (Saltin and Karlsson, 1972).

obtained just above 100 g of protein, 150−160 g of fat, and close to 400 g of carbohydrates per day.

The intake of carbohydrate well equals the normal glycogen stores of the body, and suggests that these regularly trained subjects utilize their body stores of carbohydrates during one day. In spite of the large daily intake of food, many of the athletes had a dietary intake of vitamins and iron underneath the supported daily requirements. The reason for this is that snacks (chocolate, lemonade) constitute a fairly large proportion of the daily energy (carbohydrate) intake.

DIETARY MANIPULATION TO ACHIEVE ENHANCED GLYCOGEN STORES

A special high carbohydrate diet leads to glycogen concentration in thigh musculature that is two to three times greater than normal (Bergström et al., 1967; Hultman, 1967). Figure 4 shows how a high muscle glycogen content can be achieved by varying diet and hard physical exercise. The factors that determine the magnitude of this glycogen deposit in the musculature have not yet been established (Adolfsson and Ahrén, 1971; Hultman, Bergström, and Roch-Norlund, 1971). However, experience has shown that it is impossible to attain extremely high glycogen storage in the muscles at more frequent intervals than a few weeks, even if the program in the figure is followed.

Results with special diets have been put into practice in different endurance events such as long distance skiing, running, and cycling. Even if the experience of most competitors with glycogen storage before endurance competitions was apparently favorable, a certain amount of exaggerated belief in the capability of high carbohydrate diets arose. Among other things, some people expected it to be possible for them to maintain a harder pace not just at the end of a race but from the very beginning. However, this is not the case. Filled glycogen stores only make it possible to maintain an optimal running pace (which depends upon the individual's maximal oxygen uptake and technique) from start to finish, even with exertion of very long duration (Karlsson and Saltin, 1971).

Water is bound when glycogen is stored in the liver (Puckett and Wiley, 1932). By determining body water with tritium-labeled water, it has been found that water is probably bound to glycogen when the latter is stored in skeletal musculature, and this water is released when glycogen is broken down during exercise (Koszlowski and Saltin, 1964; Saltin, 1964). When glycogen stores are filled to maximum, the water bound in this manner may amount to 2−3 liters (body weight increased by 2.5−3.5 kg) (Olsson and Saltin, 1970). The body thereby acquires a

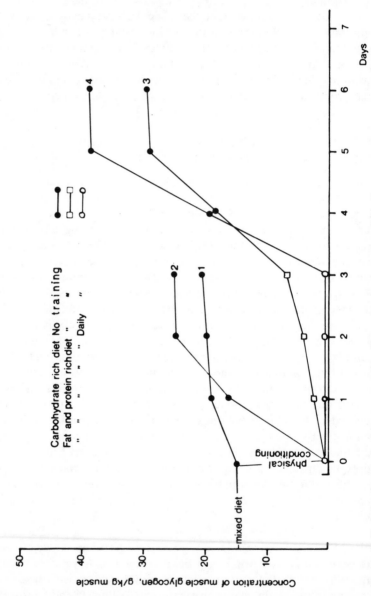

Figure 4. Variation in muscle glycogen content with acute exercise and various diets.

water reserve that can contribute to the prevention of dehydration when sweat losses rise. The decline in body weight that occurs during exercise need not indicate, therefore, any decline in functional water volume.

The stockpiling of glycogen before the start of exercise seems, therefore, to satisfy the double purpose of providing a very efficient source of energy, utilized primarily during exercise, and of providing a water reserve. It has been claimed that it takes between 2 to 3 days after completion of exercise for the body to be rehydrated (Greenleaf, 1966). It is probable that the relatively slow buildup of glycogen in the musculature (Figure 4) contributes to this. It is also essential to note that some source of food (carbohydrates) must be ingested so that normal body weight and normal water balance can be reestablished following muscular exercise of long duration.

ROLE OF FAT

The role of free fatty acids and intramuscular lipids was only touched upon briefly above. This was not because these substances are not utilized during muscular work, but because normally nourished people in well-developed countries have large energy reserves (a minimum of 2−3 kg) stored in the form of fat, and it has not been established that the administration of fat to the musculature during exercise of long duration is a limiting factor.

Recent studies have demonstrated that a substantial increase in the relative role of fat as a fuel for muscular exercise occurs with training. The training effect seems to be strictly local in nature, i.e., the muscles involved in the training obtain an enhanced oxidative potential and the augmented fat oxidation only occurs in the trained muscles (Saltin et al., 1976, Henriksson, 1977).

It has not been established to what extent work intensity in training is of significance for the reduction in the blood's concentration of lipids such as triglycerides. The background to this question is whether a special muscle fiber type activation during work is of any significance to the role regular training plays in reducing the concentration of blood lipids. In heavy exercise leading to exhaustion within 5−10 min and repeated at certain intervals, slow twitch and fast twitch fibers are activated and mainly glycogen is consumed (Gollnick, Piehl, and Saltin, 1974). The metabolic pattern with relatively heavy exertion of long duration is different; only slow twitch fibers are activated. A mobilization of free fatty acids takes place, and fatty acids and other serum lipids are taken up and oxidized in the musculature (Ahlborg, 1974; Gollnick, Piehl, and Saltin, 1974). The above could be interpreted to mean that severe intensity training, recommended as an efficient circulatory training model, is perhaps not the most appropriate form of training from the metabolic point of view. With respect to body weight, however, regardless of whether fat or carbohydrates are primarily used as the substrate in working muscle, increased caloric consumption during physical activity must invariably play a role.

ADMINISTRATION OF FLUIDS, ELECTROLYTES, AND GLUCOSE DURING ACTIVITY

The significance of food and fluid intake before severe exertion of long duration has been emphasized above. This does not mean that food and fluid administration during activity is without value. Some of the physiological considerations in relation to such an intake are now discussed.

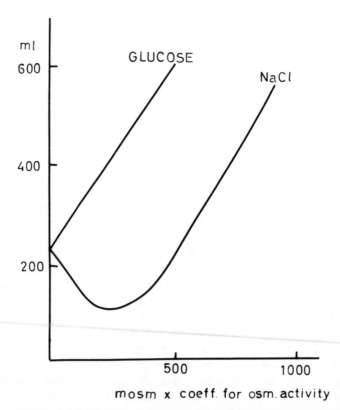

Figure 5. Volume remaining in the stomach 20 min after a test meal of 750 ml. (Adapted from Hunt and Pathak, 1960.)

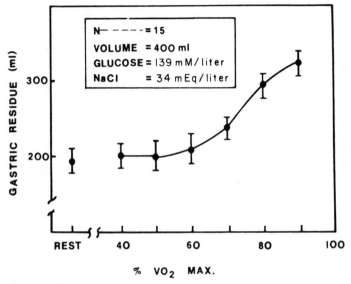

Figure 6. The effect of the intensity of the exercise for the volume remaining in the stomach 15 min after a test meal of 400 ml (Costill and Saltin, 1974).

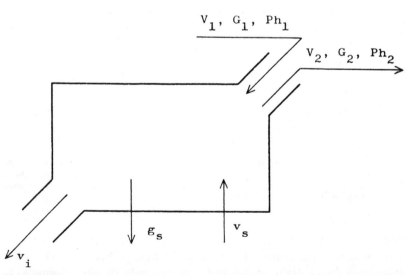

Figure 7. The model used to evaluate gastric emptying (v_i) and whether any glucose was absorbed (g_s) or water secreted (v_s) while the solution was in the stomach. Phenolred was used as an inert marker. The volume (Ph_1) of the test meal is indicated by V_1, and glucose concentration by G_1. The corresponding indices for the gastric residue are V_2, G_2, and Ph_2 (Pedersen, 1975).

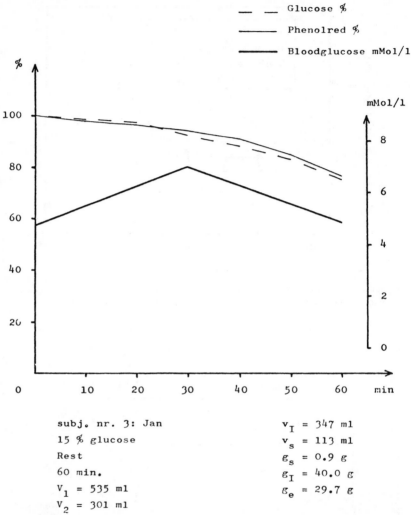

Figure 8. Typical results from an experiment with 15% glucose solution. Gastric residue and blood glucose concentration are studied at different times during 60 min of rest. Note that the glucose concentration and the phenolred concentration follow each other closely, indicating no absorption of the glucose while in the stomach (Pedersen, 1975).

Gastric Emptying

Many factors influence the emptying rate of the stomach, but here the only focus is on the osmolality. Hunt and Pathak (1960) studied in detail different solutes, their osmolality, and the rate of gastric emptying (Figure 5). Generally speaking, many solutes already at low concentration inhibit gastric emptying markedly. In absolute values, a 10% glucose concentration reduces the volume passing the stomach to half,

V_i ml

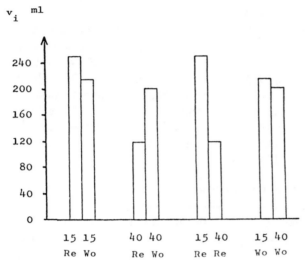

Figure 9. Value emptied to the intestine (V_i) at rest (Re) and work at 60% of V_{O_2} max for 60 min (Wo) comparing a 15 and 40% glucose solution. The interesting finding is the bar to the right indicating that a 40% glucose solution can be emptied as quickly as a 15% solution (Pedersen, 1975).

and a 40% solution of glucose is retarded to one-fifth of plain water. Hunt and Pathak (1960) have published results indicating a positive effect of NaCl at low concentrations (0.2−0.4%) on gastric emptying. Costill and Saltin (1974) have not been able to confirm this. Instead, glucose and sodium chloride have an additive effect in inhibiting the emptying of the stomach. However, the practical importance of this is minor because the need for sodium chloride is quite small, even in situations of large sweat losses.

Of greater importance are some recent observations pointing to a nonlinear relationship during exercise between increased glucose concentration and inhibition of the gastric emptying (Pedersen, 1975). Fifteen and 40% glucose concentrations were used, and at rest the values for the emptying rate followed grossly the "Hunt relationship." During exercise especially the high glucose concentration was emptied substantially faster than expected. With such a high content of glucose in the solution, only a small increase in emptying rate is of importance for the amount of glucose emptied into the intestine. In this set of experiments the exercise augmented the gastric emptying rate. This is not the typical finding. Exercise seems to have no influence at work rates of up to 70−75% of maximal oxygen uptake (heart rate ≈ 160 beats/min), but above that, exercise intensity moderately inhibited the rate of stomach emptying (Figure 6).

Absorption of Solutes by the Stomach

The studies described with 15 and 40% glucose solutions were performed with the primary aim of studying glucose and water absorption while the solution was in the stomach. Some of the results are depicted in Figures 7, 8, and 9. No significant uptake of either glucose or water could be detected during the one hour the experiments lasted. This is in accordance with previous studies (Fordtran and Saltin, 1967). In some studies sodium chloride was also included in the solution, but it did not affect the uptake of water and glucose, and no uptake of the sodium chloride could be observed.

Absorption in the Intestine

Up to an exercise intensity of around 70% of maximal oxygen uptake, no significant change in the magnitude of the absorption of water, sodium, potassium, chloride, and glucose by different parts of the in-

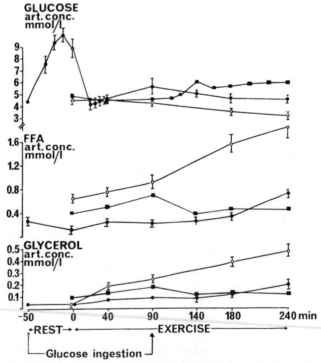

Figure 10. Arterial concentration for glucose, FFA, and glycerol in three different series of experiments. Each experiment consisted of a rest period (50 min) and exercise for 240 min at 30% V_{O_2} max. In one series no glucose was given (O), and in the other two, 200 g of glucose were administered either 50 min before (●) the exercise or after (■) 90 min of exercise. (Adapted from Ahlborg and Fehlig, 1977.)

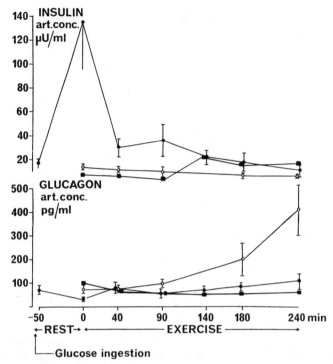

Figure 11.   Arterial insulin and glucagon concentration in the three conditions mentioned in Figure 10. (Adapted from Ahlborg and Fehlig, 1977.)

testine could be detected (Fordtran and Saltin, 1967). Above this exercise intensity no complete studies are available, but some using radioactive labeled glucose do indicate that it is absorbed, because significant amounts of specific activity for the isotope are found both in blood and expired CO_2 (Costill et al., 1973).

Effects on the Body

The fate of water and electrolytes within the body, absorbed from the gut during exercise, is largely unknown. From a theoretical standpoint, water and ions ought to equilibrate with the different fluid compartments reasonably fast because blood flow is kept at a high level and perfuses large volumes of tissues, which otherwise are only sparsely perfused. That this is the case is uncertain. It is a common finding that after many hours of severe exercise with a large but insufficient fluid intake (body weight is reduced), blood volume is increased as plasma volume is enlarged by half a liter (Åstrand and Saltin, 1964; Shepherd, personal communication). Assuming an equal distribution between intravascular and interstitial fluid compartments, the extracellular vol-

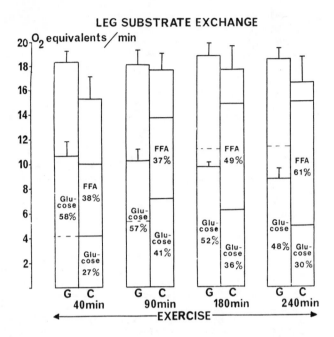

Figure 12. An estimate of the substrate exchange in the leg at different time intervals during exercise in the control and the glucose experiments. Note the thin dashed line in the bars of the glucose experiments, indicating the results from the experiments when the glucose was given after 90 min of exercise. (Adapted from Ahlborg and Fehlig, 1977.)

ume may be expanded 1–2 liters, in spite of a lowered body weight of the same magnitude. It is true that water liberated from the metabolic processes, including the water presumably liberated when glycogen is utilized, may be part of the explanation. However, it is difficult to believe that this is the whole answer. Further study is indeed needed for a more complete understanding of fluid regulation of the body while exercising.

Until recently the knowledge about the effects of glucose administration in connection with exercise was not studied in any detail in man. Ahlborg and Felig (1977a,b) have recently completed two studies: in one, 200 g of glucose was given orally (saturated solution, 50 min before a 4-hr exercise period at 30–35% of maximal oxygen uptake), and in the other study the same amount was given after 90 min of exercise (Figure 10–12).

Both the splanchnic output and the leg uptake of glucose were studied. With an intake of glucose before work, blood glucose and insulin were initially high during the exercise and remained elevated throughout the exercise period. The utilization of glucose by the leg was also higher and the R-values were elevated. This larger use of extra

muscular carbohydrate was matched by an enlarged release of glucose from the splanchnic area without any increase in the gluconeogenesis. When the glucose was given after 1½ hr of exercise, arterial glucose and insulin levels became elevated within 30 min and remained so until the end of the experiments. Again the exercising muscles increased their uptake of glucose from the bloodstream, and it was matched by the output of glucose from the splanchnic area. Glucagon, which usually is increased markedly in prolonged exercise, remained unchanged, and so did the uptake of glucose metabolites. The results of these two studies demonstrate clearly that glucose given orally in connection with prolonged exercise is utilized during the work period. The R-values suggest an enlarged total carbohydrate metabolism, which means that muscle glycogen may not have been saved. In the liver, the synthesis of glucose from gluconeogenic substances declined. Whether a lowering of the carbohydrate store in the liver occurs or not cannot be settled. In fact, it may have been increased, because far from all of the injected glucose appeared in the arterial blood.

REFERENCES

Adolfsson, S., and Ahrén, K. 1971. Control mechanisms for the synthesis of glycogen in striated muscle. In B. Pernow and B. Saltin (eds.), Muscle Metabolism During Exercise, p. 257–272. Plenum Press, New York.

Adolph, E. F. 1947. Physiology of Man in the Desert. Interscience Publishers, New York.

Ahlborg, G. 1974. Glucose Metabolism in Exercising Man. Thesis, Karolinska Institutet, Stockholm.

Ahlborg, G., and Felig, P. 1977. Substrate utilization during prolonged exercise preceded by ingestion of glucose. Am. J. Physiol. 233: 188.

Ahlborg, G., and Felig, P. 1976. Influence of glucose ingestion on the fuel-hormone response during prolonged exercise. J. Appl. Physiol. 41: 683.

Åstrand, P.-O., and Saltin, B. 1964. Plasma and red cell volume after prolonged severe exercise. J. of Appl. Physiol. 19: 829.

Barr, P.-O, Birke, G., Liljedahl, S.-O, and Plantin, L.-O. 1968. Oxygen consumption and water loss during treatment of burns with warm dry air. Lancet i: 164.

Bergström, J., Hermansen, L., Hultman, E., and Saltin, B. 1967. Diet, muscle glycogen and physical performance. Acta Physiol. Scand. 71: 140.

Blix, G. 1965. A study on the relation between total calories and single nutrients in food. Acta Soc. Med. Upsalien 70: 17.

Bonnesen, A., and Rasmussen, I. B. 1976. Begraensende faktorer for arbejdskapaciteten ved et meget hardt arbejde. (Factors limiting work capacity after prolonged intense exercise.) Report no. 100, August Krogh Institute, Copenhagen.

Buskirk, E. R., Iampietro, R. F., and Bass, D. E. 1958. Work performance after dehydration. Effects of physical conditioning and heat acclimatization. J. Appl. Physiol. 12: 189.

Costill, D. L., Bennett, A., Broman, G., and Eddy, D. 1973. Glucose ingestion at rest and during prolonged exercise. J. Appl. Physiol. 34: 764.

Costill, D. L., and Saltin, B. 1974. Factors limiting gastric emptying during rest and exercise. J. Appl. Physiol. 37: 679–683.

Ekelund, L.-G. 1967. Circulatory and respiratory adaptation during prolonged exercise. Acta Physiol. Scand. (suppl.): 292.

Felig, P., Pozefsky, T., Marliss, E., and Cahill, G. F., Jr. 1970. Alanine: Key role in gluconeogenesis. Science 167: 1003.

Felig, P., and Wahren, V. 1971a. Interrelationship between amino acid and carbohydrate metabolism during exercise: The glucose alanine cycle. In: B. Pernow and B. Saltin (eds.), Muscle Metabolism During Exercise, pp. 205–214. Plenum Press, New York.

Felig, P., and Wahren, J. 1971b. Amino acid metabolism in exercising man. J. Clin. Invest. 50: 2703.

Fordtran, J. S., and Saltin, B. 1967. Gastric emptying and intestinal absorption during prolonged severe exercise. J. Appl. Physiol. 23: 331.

Gollnick, P. D., Piehl, K, and Saltin, B. 1974. Selective depletion patterns in human muscle fibers after varying intensity and at varying pedalling rates. J. Physiol. 241: 45–51.

Greenleaf, J. E. 1966. Involuntary hypohydration in man and animals. A review, NASA, S P-110, Washington, D. C.

Henriksson, J. 1976. Human skeletal muscle adaptation to physical activity. Thesis. Karolinska Institutet, Stockholm.

Hermansen, L., Hultman, E., and Saltin, B. 1967. Muscle glycogen during prolonged severe exercise. Acta Physiol. Scand. 71: 129.

Hultman, E. 1967. Studies on muscle metabolism of glycogen and active phosphate in man with special reference to exercise and diet. Scand. J. Clin. Lab. Invest. 19 (suppl.): 94.

Hultman, E., Bergstrom, J., and Roch-Norlund, A. E. 1971. Glycogen storage in human skeletal muscle. In B. Pernow and B. Saltin (eds.), Muscle Metabolism During Exercise, pp. 273–288. Plenum Press, New York.

Hultman, E., and Nilsson, L. H:son, 1971. Liver glycogen in man: Effect of different diets and muscular exercise. In B. Pernow and B. Saltin (eds.), Muscle Metabolism During Exercise, pp. 143–152. Plenum Press, New York.

Hunt, J. N., and Pathak, J. O. 1960. The osmotic effects of some simple molecules and ions on gastric emptying. J. Physiol. (London) 154: 254.

Karlsson, J., and Saltin, B. 1971. Diet, muscle glycogen and endurance performance. J. Appl. Physiol. 31: 203–206.

Koszlowski, S., and Saltin, B. 1964. Effect of sweat loss on body fluids. J. Appl. Physiol. 19: 1119–1124.

Kuno, Y. 1956. Human Perspiration. Charles C Thomas, Springfield.

Lundvall, J., Mellander, S., Westling, H., and White, T. 1972. Fluid transfer between blood and tissues during exercise. Acta Physiol. Scand. 85: 258–269.

Malette, L. E., Exton, J. H., and Park, C. R. 1969. Control of gluconeogenesis from various procursors in the perfused rat liver. Biochem. J. 102: 942.

Nielsen, M. 1938. Die Regulation der Körpertemperatur bei Muskelarbeit. (The regulation of body temperature during muscular work.) Skand. Arch. Physiol. 79: 193.

Nishi, Y., and Gagge, A. P. 1970. Direct evaluation of convective heat transfer coefficient by naphthalene sublimation. J. Appl. Physiol. 29: 830.

Olsson, K.-E., and Saltin, B. 1970. Variation in total body water with muscle glycogen changes in man. Acta Physiol. Scand. 80: 11.

Pedersen, E. F. 1975. Staerke glucoseopløsnigers virkning pa mavesaekkens optagelse af glucose, pa legemets vaeskeudbytte og pa blodglucosekoncentrationen, i hvile og under arbejde. (Glucose uptake in the stomach.) Report no. 79. August Krogh Institute, Copenhagen.

Puckett, H. L., and Wiley, F. H. 1932. The relation of glycogen to water storage in the liver. J. Biol. Chem. 96: 367–371.

Robinson, S., and Robinson, A. H. 1954. Chemical composition of sweat. Physiol. Rev. 34: 202–220.

Rosell, S., and Saltin, B. 1973. Energy need and utilization in exercise. In Bourne (ed.), Muscle, Vol. 3. Academic Press, New York.

Rowell, L. B. 1971. The liver as an energy source in man during exercise. In B. Pernow and B. Saltin (eds.), Muscle Metabolism During Exercise, pp. 127–14. Plenum Press, New York.

Rowell, L. B., Kranig, K. K., III, Evans, T. O., Kennedy, J. W., Blackmon, J. R., and Kusami, F. 1966. Splanchnic removal of lactate and puruvate during prolonged exercise in man. J. Appl. Physiol. 21: 1773.

Rowell, L. B., Masoro, E. J., and Spencer, M. J. 1965. Splanchnic metabolism in exercising man. J. Appl. Physiol. 20: 1032.

Saltin, B. 1964. Aerobic work capacity and circulation at exercise in man. Acta Physiol. Scand. 62(suppl.):230.

Saltin, B. 1964. Aerobic and anaerobic work capacity after dehydration. J. Appl. Physiol. 19: 1114–1118.

Saltin, B., Gagge, A. P., and Stolwijk, J. A. J. 1968. Muscle temperature during submaximal exercise in man. J. Appl. Physiol. 25: 679–688.

Saltin, B., Gagge, A. P., and Stolwijk, J. A. J. 1970. Body temperatures and sweating during thermal transients caused by exercise. J. Appl. Physiol. 28: 318–327.

Saltin, B., and Hermansen, L. 1966. Esophageal, rectal and muscle temperature during exercise. J. Appl. Physiol. 21: 1757.

Saltin, B., and Hermansen, L. 1967. Glycogen stores and prolonged severe exercise. In G. Blix (ed.), Symposia of the Swedish Nutrition Foundation V, p. 32. Almqvist and Wiksell, Stockholm.

Saltin, B., and Karlsson, J. 1971. Muscle ATP, CP, and lactate during exercise after physical conditioning. In B. Pernow and B. Saltin (eds.), Muscle Metabolism During Exercise, pp. 395–399. Plenum Press, New York.

Saltin, B. and Karlsson, J. 1972. Die Ernährung des Sportlers. (Nutrition of sportsmen.) In Hollman (ed.), Zentrale Thema der Sportphysiologie. (Principal Topics of Sport Physiology.) Springer, Heidelberg.

Saltin, B., Nazar, K., Costill, D. L., Stein, E, Jansson, E., Essen, B., and Gollnick, P. D. 1976. The nature of the training response; Peripheral and central adaptations to one-legged exercise. Acta Physiol. Scand. 96: 289–305.

Saltin, B., and Stenberg, J. 1965. Circulatory response to prolonged severe exercise. J. Appl. Physiol. 20: 833–838.

Snellen, J. O. 1966. Mean body temperature and the control of thermal sweating. Acta Physiol. Scand. Pharma. Neerl. 14: 99–174.

Stolwijk, J. A. J., Saltin, B., and Gagge, A. P. 1968. Physiological factors associated with sweating during exercise. Aerospace Med. 39: 1100.

Vellar, O. 1969. Nutrient losses through sweating. Thesis. Oslo.

Wahren, J., Ahlborg, G., Felig, P., and Jorfeldt, L. 1971. Glucose metabolism during exercise in man. In B. Pernow and B. Saltin (eds.), Muscle Metabolism During Exercise, pp. 189–203. Plenum Press, New York.

Wretlind, A. 1968. Nutrition problems in healthy adults with low activity and low caloric consumption. In G. Blix (ed.), Occurrence, Causes, and Prevention of Nutritional-Anemias, p. 114. Almqvist and Wiksell, Uppsala. 1967.

Muscle Water and Electrolytes During Acute and Repeated Bouts of Dehydration

D. L. Costill

It is well documented that large sweat losses can dramatically impair the performance of endurance athletes (Åstrand and Saltin, 1964; Saltin, 1964a; Costill, Kammer, and Fisher, 1970). Because decrements in performance are generally thought to be the result of a diminished circulatory capacity, it is no surprise that physiologists have concentrated their research on the cardiovascular responses of acutely dehydrated man. It is, in fact, generally agreed that a sweat loss constituting more than 2% of body weight can significantly reduce plasma volume and impair physical work capacity (Saltin, 1964b; Costill and Sparks, 1973).

Traditionally, studies of body fluid distribution in acutely dehydrated man have been limited to indirect dilution measurements of plasma, interstitial, and intracellular volumes (Kozlowski and Saltin, 1964; Costill and Fink, 1974). Although such studies have partially described the distribution of body water losses, they fail to define the significance of sweat and urine electrolyte losses on muscle tissue fluids.

The purpose of the following discussion, therefore, is to describe the changes in muscle water and electrolytes following acute and repeated bouts of dehydration. Specific attention is given to the following topics: 1) the effects of varied levels of dehydration, 2) changes in active and inactive muscles during prolonged exertion, 3) the effects of repeated days of dehydration, and 4) the combined influence of dehydration and low dietary potassium (K^+) on muscle water and electrolytes. Attempts are made to describe the distribution of water and electrolyte

This research was supported by the National Institutes of Health (AM 17083-02). Presented at the International Symposium on Sportsmen's Nutrition in Warsaw, Poland, October 22–24, 1975.

losses on the contents of plasma, interstitial, and intracellular fluids. The water lost in sweat is generally proportional to the subject's body surface area, rate of energy expenditure, and the thermal nature of the environment. As one might anticipate, the slope of the regression depicted in Figure 1 will shift to the left with increasing environmental heat (Costill, Kammer, and Fisher, 1970). As a result, body water losses following prolonged exercise may exceed 6 liters, constituting nearly 10% of the subject's body weight. Because the body is roughly 60% water, a 6-liter sweat loss may decrease a 65 kg runner's body water content by about 15%.

The ionic concentration of sweat may vary markedly between individuals and is strongly affected by the rate of sweating and heat acclimatization. In general, however, the Na^+, K^+, Cl^-, and Mg^{++} concentrations in sweat are similar to those listed in Table 1. It is apparent that the principal ions of sweat are those of the extracellular

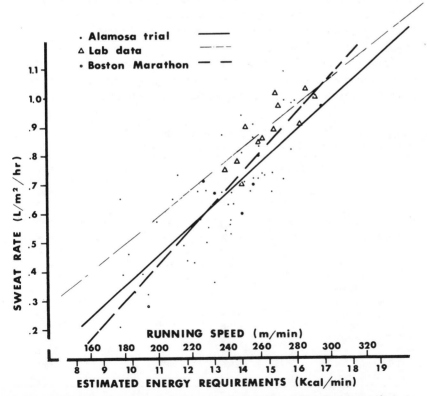

Figure 1. Relationship between running speed (energy expenditure) and sweating rate during treadmill (2 hr) and marathon running.

compartment, namely Na^+ and Cl^-. As a point of reference, it should be noted that the total NaCl lost during the 5.8% dehydration is roughtly 6 to 8% of the total exchangeable Na^+ and Cl^- in the body (Figure 2). The relatively small K^+ and Mg^{++} losses, on the other hand, constitute only about 1% of the body stores.

VARIED LEVELS OF DEHYDRATION

In an effort to examine the changes in muscle water and electrolytes resulting from varying degrees of dehydration, eight men were studied before and after weight losses of 2.2, 4.1, and 5.8%. Sweating was promoted by continuous cycling exercise at 60−70% of Vo_2 max in an environmental chamber maintained at 39° C with a relative humidity of 25%.

Blood (venous), muscle (vastus lateralis), sweat (wash down method), and urine measurements were made before and at the completion of each level of dehydration (Bergström 1962; Vellar, 1968; Dill and Costill, 1974). Losses of extra- and intracellular water and electrolytes were calculated as previously described by Bergström (1962) and Costill, Coté, and Fink (1976).

Because the major ions lost in sweat and urine were those of the extracellular compartment, it is not surprising to observe a disproportionately larger loss of water from plasma and interstitial spaces than

Table 1.   Concentration of Na^+, K^+, Cl^-, and Mg^{++} in sweat of men and women during 90 min of intermittent and continuous exercise in the heat[a]

	Sweat rate	Sweat ions (mEq/liter)			
	(liters/hr)	Na^+	K^+	Cl^-	Mg^{++}
Males (N = 12)					
Intermittent (75% Vo_2 max)	1.28 (±0.10)	50.9 (±3.8)	4.4 (±0.2)	42.9 (±3.1)	2.5 (±0.4)
Continuous (53% Vo_2 max)	1.36 (±0.10)	39.2 (±4.0)	4.2 (±0.2)	34.9 (±3.3)	1.6 (±0.3)
Females (N = 12)					
Intermittent (75% Vo_2 max)	0.55 (±.04)	38.8 (±5.6)	5.0 (±0.2)	30.3 (±4.5)	4.3 (±1.4)
Continuous (53% Vo_2 max)	0.60 (±.04)	42.4 (±8.6)	4.6 (±0.3)	39.1 (±3.6)	4.9 (±1.6)

[a] 35°C, 20% relative humidity. Total energy requirements for the two exercise conditions were equal. Values represent the means (±SE).

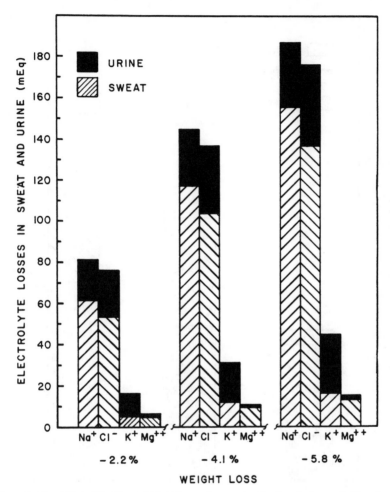

Figure 2. Total Na$^+$, K$^+$, Cl$^-$ and Mg^{++} losses in sweat and urine during varied levels of dehydration.

from the intracellular compartment. Although plasma and interstitial water declined approximately 2.5% for each percent of dehydration, the intracellular water decreased only 1.1% for each percent of dehydration. The absolute loss of water from these compartments, however, was quite evenly distributed between the extra- and intracellular spaces (Figure 3). It is interesting to note that at all stages of dehydration, plasma water accounts for 10–11% of the total body water loss. Except for the 2.2% stage of dehydration, intracellular fluids contribute roughly half of the water lost.

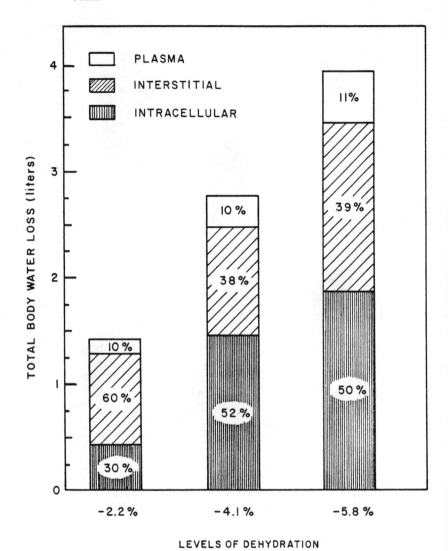

Figure 3. Distribution of water lost from plasma, interstitial, and intracellular compartments during varied levels of dehydration.

In keeping with the previous calculations of the change in intracellular water, muscle water declined steadily with dehydration (Table 2). This change constituted a 6.8% decrease in muscle water, which is similar to the change in intracellular water (-6.5%) determined by the loss of Cl^- in urine and sweat. The values reported in Table 2 for muscle Na^+, K^+, and Cl^- content were not statistically significant at any stage of dehydration. Only muscle Mg^{++} content showed a significant change, decreasing 12% following the final stage of dehydration (-5.8%).

These values are computed on the basis of the fat-free solid weight of the tissue, so they do not reflect the concentration of the ions in muscle water. As a result of the decline in muscle water, the ions present in the tissue samples were concentrated. Thus, the K^+_i increased significantly, but Mg^{++}_i and Na^+_i remained unchanged.

Based on the preceding data and the equation by Hodgkin and Horowicz (1959), it is possible to estimate what effects dehydration might have on the muscle's resting membrane potential. It was estimated that the resting muscle membrane potential (RMP) averaged -91.4 mV before dehydration and remained unchanged at all levels of body weight loss (Johns, 1960; Cunningham et al., 1971). Although such methods of determining the RMP must be viewed cautiously, these calculations confirm earlier studies and suggest that dehydration does not alter the excitability of the muscle cell membrane (Costill and Saltin, 1975).

Thus, this series of observations demonstrates that body water lost during acute dehydration is attributed to relatively larger water losses from extracellular than from intracellular compartments. Despite large sweat losses, the muscle K^+ content remained unchanged, but increased in concentration as a result of the loss of water from the muscle tissue. However, one should not overlook the fact that these measurements were made following 30 min of rest, and muscle samples were obtained only from a heavily exercised muscle.

ACTIVE VERSUS INACTIVE MUSCLES

One might ask, "how representative is the exercising m. vastus lateralis of other less active muscles?" In an effort to answer this

Table 2.   Muscle water, electrolytes, and glycogen content before and after varied degrees of dehydration

	Per 100 g fat-free solids					
Dehydration	H_2O_m (ml)	Na^+_m (mEq)	K^+_m (mEq)	Cl^-_m (mEq)	Mg^{++}_m (mEq)	Glycogen (mmole/kg)
0	341	9.9	46.3	6.1	9.0	115
-2.2%	329	10.4	47.4	6.6	8.3	76
-4.1%	324	11.1	47.0	8.3	8.1	61
-5.8%	318	9.6	47.8	6.2	7.9	48

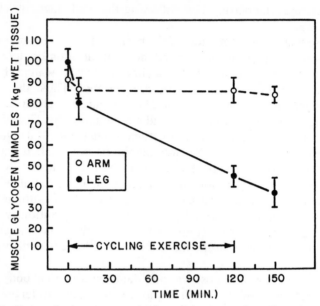

Figure 4. Changes in glycogen content of exercising (vastus lateralis) and nonexercising (deltoid) muscles during 2 hr of cycling.

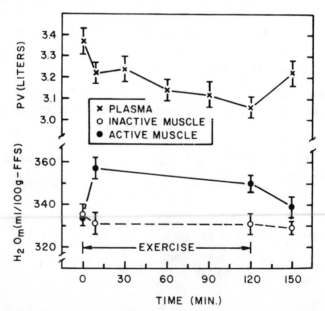

Figure 5. Changes in plasma volume and water content of inactive (deltoid) and active (vastus lateralis) muscles during 2 hr of cycling.

query, seven men were studied before, during, and after 2 hr of exercise at roughly 60% Vo_2 max. Muscle biopsies were obtained from exercising (vastus lateralis) and nonexercising (deltoid) muscles before, at 10 and 120 min of cycling, and after 30 min of recovery from the activity. Venous blood was sampled before and after 10, 30, 60, 90, and 120 min of exercise and assayed for selected ions (K^+, Na^+, Cl^-, and Mg^{++}), as well as for changes in water content. Muscle specimens were subsequently analyzed for water, electrolytes, and glycogen content as previously described (Bergström, 1962). As shown in Figure 4, the glycogen content of the vastus lateralis decreased 64 mmole/kg wet tissue as a result of the exercise, but the glycogen in the deltoid (inactive muscle) remained unchanged.

The combined loss of body water via sweating, respiration, and urination produced a 3.2% reduction in body weight. Electrolyte excretion (sweat plus urine) during this period averaged 92.6 mEq Na^+, 22.3 mEq K^+, 94.8 mEq Cl^-, and 4.6 mEq Mg^{++}. These values confirm the fact that relatively little K^+ and Mg^{++} is lost during prolonged exercise.

At the onset of exercise, plasma volume decreased 4.4%. This loss of water from plasma is apparently the result of a transcapillary fluid flux in the exercising muscle (Figure 5). Muscle tissue taken from the thigh showed a 6.8% increase in water content, but the water in the inactive muscle remained unchanged. This movement of water into the active tissues is the result of an increase in hydrostatic pressure and a

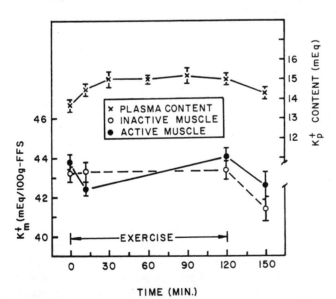

Figure 6. Changes in the K^+ content of plasma (K^+_p), exercising muscles (vastus lateralis), and inactive muscles (deltoid) during exercise and recovery.

tissue hyperosmolality (Kjellmer, 1964; Mellander et al., 1967). This difference in the H_2O content of active and inactive tissues persists throughout the 2-hr exercise bout despite a gradual decline in plasma volume (Figure 5).

In the early minutes of muscular activity, there is an efflux of K^+ from the cell (Miller and Darrow, 1941; Costill and Saltin, 1975) (Figure 6). Subsequently, exercise-dehydration seems to have little effect on the plasma K^+ content, but K^+ seemed to re-enter the active muscles.

Exercising muscle seems to slowly increase its Mg^{++} content, which is paralleled by a gradual decline in plasma. This Mg^{++} movement into contracting muscle is a function of the increased metabolic need. Unfortunately, these data do not permit one to detail the mechanism responsible for this change or its physiological significance.

Thus, it seems that there are marked differences between active and inactive muscles with regard to their water and ionic contents during both short-term and prolonged exercise. During the first 30 min of recovery, however, these constituents are redistributed so that both tissues have similar water and electrolyte contents. Therefore, muscle tissues sampled from a single site can be used to estimate the effects of dehydration on muscle water and electrolytes, providing the subject has been inactive for 30 min. These observations also suggest that attempts to calculate the distribution of muscle water and ions by the choloride method may be invalidated by a shift in the membrane potential.

REPEATED DAYS OF EXERCISE AND DEHYDRATION

To this point the acute effects of exercise and large sweat losses on muscle fluids have been considered. Although there have been some marked changes noted in muscle ions and water during exercise, the principal effect of acute dehydration is in reducing muscle water with little influence on the muscle Na^+, K^+, Cl^-, and Mg^{++} content. As a result, one is led to conclude that aside from the temporary loss of body water, ions lost in sweat probably have little effect on their function in muscle. It has been suggested, however, that individuals who perform heavy exercise and who sweat profusely on repeated days may incur deficits of selected ions, principally K^+ (Saltin, 1964a; Knochel, Dotin, and Hamburger, 1972). Despite many accusations, no direct evidence of tissue hypokalemia has been provided to substantiate these claims.

The author attempted to gain some insight into this problem by studying 12 subjects (10 men, 2 women) during five successive days of dehydration (Costill et al., 1975). Although the subjects were permitted to eat and drink ad libitum, the total water, K^+, Na^+, Cl^-, and caloric intake was closely monitored. Likewise, the daily excretion of water and ions in sweat and urine were accurately measured. These body water and electrolyte exchange data revealed that repeated days of exercise-dehydration induced a renal conservation of Na^+ with a small decline in urine K^+. As a result, the subjects tended to store Na^+ (392 mEq/5 days), while total body K^+ increased roughly 100 mEq during the five days of these observations. The relatively large gains in Na^+ were accompanied by a proportionate increase in extracellular water. This is well documented by the expansion of plasma volume illustrated in Figure 7. It is interesting to note that 48 to 72 hr were required for the elimination of this "excess" water and extracellular ion.

The mechanism apparently responsible for this Na^+ conserving response to successive days of dehydration is an increase in mineral corticoid function. Exposure to heat, exercise, and/or dehydration results in arterial hypovolemia and relative renal ischemia. Both factors are known to be responsible for increased aldosterone production and renal sodium reabsorption (Bartter and Gann, 1960; Hartroft and Hartroft, 1961). This point is documented by changes in plasma renin and aldosterone concentrations following a single bout (1 hr) of exercise (Figure 8). Despite ad libitum water intake, plasma aldosterone remains elevated for nearly 12 hr following such exercise.

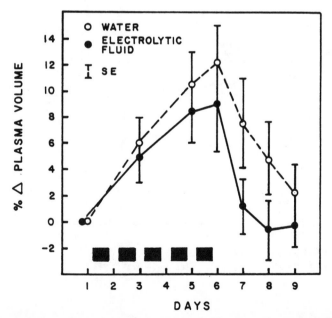

Figure 7. Percentage change in plasma volume during five days of repeated dehydration (−3% per day). During one series the subjects were only permitted to drink water, but in the second treatment thirst was satisfied by ad libitum ingestion of an electrolyte drink.

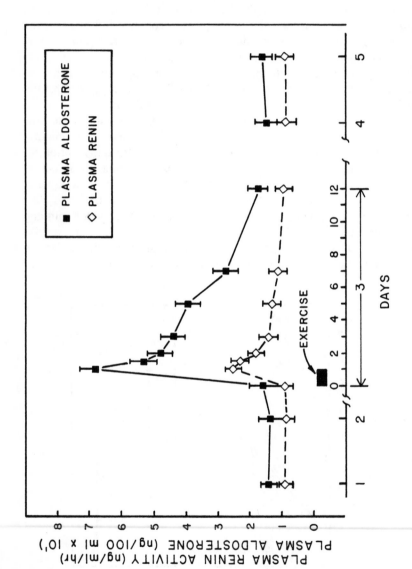

Figure 8. Alterations in plasma renin activity and aldosterone concentration as a result of a single 60-min exercise bout.

Thus, despite the sweat and urinary losses incurred during dehydration, men and women can maintain a positive Na^+, K^+, and Cl^- balance via dietary intake and renal conservation of these ions, on the condition that food and drink are provided ad libitum. Nevertheless, it has been suggested that under some occupational and athletic situations it is possible for persons to lose more than 6–8% of body weight by heavy sweating, with Na^+ and K^+ losses in excess of 200 and 40 mEq/24 hr, respectively. Although such loss provides strong stimuli for renal Na^+ conservation, it is possible that the kidney may continue to excrete K^+ despite a serious body potassium deficit.

Knochel, Dotin, and Hamburger (1972) observed that six men undergoing intensive physical training in a hot climate developed a mean K^+ deficit of 349 mEq in the first four days of exercise. This deficit, estimated from measurements of $[^{42}K]$, occurred despite a daily K^+ intake of 100 mEq/day. Unfortunately, the balance of K^+ intake and excretion (sweat, urine, and feces) was not adequately monitored to validate the $[^{42}K]$ calculations. If, in fact, heavy sweating and exercise

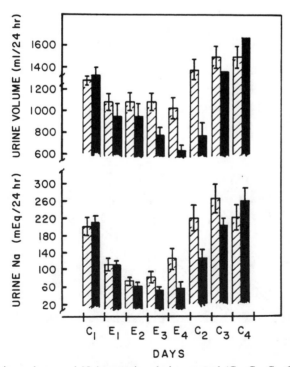

Figure 9. Urine volume and Na^+ excretion during control (C_1, C_2, C_3, C_4) and four repeated days of exercise (E_1–E_4). Hashed vertical bars represent values during the high K^+ diet (80 mEq/24 hr), and solid bars denote urine values during the low K^+ diet (25 mEq/24 hr).

on repeated days can induce such large body K^+ deficits, then such changes should be detectable in muscle biopsy specimens.

For that reason, an investigation was recently conducted to determine the effects of low dietary K^+ and repeated days of heavy exercise on muscle water and electrolytes. Eight men exercised sufficiently on four successive days to achieve a mean body weight loss of 3.1 kg (4.2% of body weight). This protocol was followed under two dietary regimens. One diet sequence provided 25 mEq of K^+ daily (low K^+ diet), and the second contained 80 mEq of K^+ each day (high K^+ diet). Both experimental diets included 180 mEq of Na^+/day with an average daily caloric content of 2,880 kcal.

In response to the four days of exercise-dehydration, urine production decreased from a control value of approximately 1,300 ml/24 hr to a low of 600 ml/24 hr during the low K^+ dietary sequence (Figure 9). Although urine volume was depressed in both experimental treatments, the low K^+ diet elicited a significantly greater reduction than did the high K^+ diet. At the same time, there was a marked reduction in urine Na^+ excretion, which also seemed to be more pronounced during the low K^+ experiment (Figure 9). As a matter of fact, some individuals excreted less than 10 mEq of Na^+ in a 24-hr period. These patterns of reduced renal water and Na^+ excretion are similar to earlier observa-

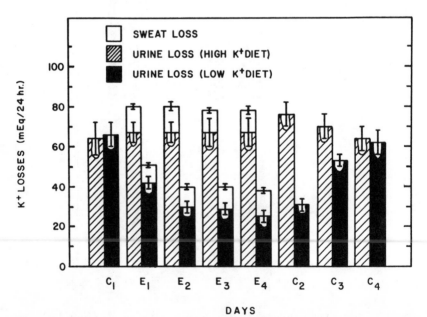

Figure 10. Sweat and urine K^+ losses during control (C_1-C_4) and repeated days of exercise (E_1-E_4). Hashed vertical bars represent values obtained during the high K^+ diet. Solid bars denote values during the low K^+ diet.

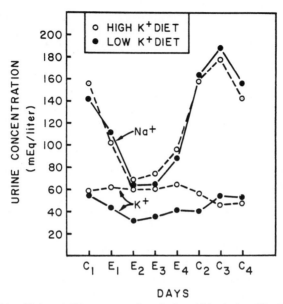

Figure 11. Urine Na$^+$ and K$^+$ concentrations before (C$_1$), during (E$_1$–E$_2$), and after (C$_2$–C$_4$) repeated days of exercise-dehydration.

tions and suggest that dietary K$^+$ may be influential in the renal Na$^+$ – water conservation during repeated days of heavy exercise (Costill et al., 1975).

Of greater interest was the rate of body K$^+$ lost in urine and sweat during the exercise and dietary regimens. As can be observed in Figure 10, there was substantially less K$^+$ excreted in urine during the low K$^+$ diet than when the men consumed the 80 mEq of K$^+$ daily. Changes in dietary K$^+$ intake had no effect on sweat K$^+$ content. If this lower renal K$^+$ excretion were a function of the reduced urine volume, then one would expect to see a decreased K$^+$ excretion in both dietary treatments and no change in the concentration of K$^+$ in urine. Figure 11 shows that urine K$^+$ concentration decreased significantly during the low K$^+$ intake, but remained relatively constant during the high K$^+$ treatment. Thus, with a reduced K$^+$ intake and repeated days of dehydration, there is a selective reduction in renal K$^+$ excretion. The mechanism responsible for this apparent K$^+$ conservation is not easily explained, but may simply reflect the lower K$^+$ entry into plasma following the low K$^+$ diet.

Thus, given the dietary intake and losses (urine and sweat) of Na$^+$ and K$^+$, it is possible to approximate the average daily change in body content (Table 3). Despite heavy sweating and relatively normal urine K$^+$ losses, the subjects were able to remain in positive K$^+$ balance with

Table 3. Average daily Na⁺ and K⁺ balance during successive days of dehydration

Type of diet		Intake (mEq/day)	Loss (mEq/day)		Balance (±mEq/day)
			Urine	Sweat	
K⁺	(high K⁺ diet)	79.9 (±2.8)	−67.1 (±4.1)	−11.5 (±0.7)	+1.3
	(low K⁺ diet)	25.0 (±0.1)	−31.7 (±3.5)	−10.4 (±0.6)	−17.1
Na⁺	(high K⁺ diet)	179.0 (±5.7)	−92.6 (±12.2)	−84.0 (±9.7)	+2.4
	(low K⁺ diet)	181.2 (±7.2)	−69.0 (±14.0)	−82.7 (±7.7)	+29.5

an intake of 80 mEq per day. When the diet contained only 25 mEq of K⁺ per day, however, the subjects incurred a body K⁺ deficit of about 17 mEq/day (−68 mEq/4 days). If we assume that these men had total body K⁺ contents of 3,450 mEq (42 mEq/kg), then the deficits incurred in this study were roughly 2% of the body K⁺ stores.

As anticipated, the subjects showed a positive Na⁺ balance during both dietary-exercise regimens, with the low K⁺ diet producing a significantly greater increase in body Na⁺ content than was observed in the high K⁺ treatment (Table 3). In light of these findings, it would seem that when combined with chronic exercise, a low K⁺ intake re-

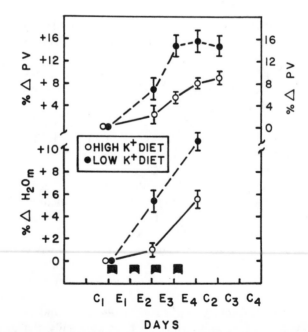

Figure 12. Percentage changes in plasma volume and muscle water content before, during, and following repeated days of exercise-dehydration. Black bars in the lower panel denote the four days of activity (E_1–E_4).

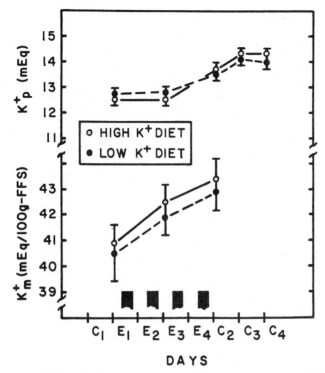

Figure 13. Alterations in the K^+ content of plasma (K^+_p) and muscle tissue (K^+_m) before, during, and after repeated days (E_1-E_4) of exercise-dehydration. Data are presented in conjunction with the low and high potassium diets.

sults in a greater aldosterone response followed by an increased rate of Na^+ and water retention.

This concept is supported by the data in Figure 12, which shows a significantly greater increase in plasma volume during the low K^+ diets than when the subjects consumed 80 mEq of K^+ each day. Muscle biopsy samples obtained at rest on the first, third, and fifth days of the experiments revealed an increase in muscle water content (H_2O_m) during both dietary conditions. In keeping with the plasma volume and Na^+ balance data, H_2O_m increased significantly more during the low K^+ diet than with the high K^+ intake.

Because the subjects showed little gain in body K^+ content ($+5$ mEq/4 days) during the high K^+ treatment and a 2% body K^+ deficit in the low K^+ experiment, it is surprising to observe the significant increase in muscle K^+ content (K^+_m) shown in Figure 13. At present this response has no explanation, but similar patterns have been observed among competitive cyclists who perform 100 km rides on four successive days. In any event, there is no evidence to support the concept that heavy exercise on repeated days will threaten the muscle and plasma K^+ stores.

Some investigators have suggested that athletes engaged in heavy training may be more susceptible to heat stress injuries as a result of depleted body K^+ stores (Schamadan and Snively, 1967; Rose, 1975). Before and after the experiments with low and high K^+ diets and repeated days of exercise, the subjects performed a 90-min heat tolerance test. Aside from excreting a more dilute sweat, all thermal (skin and rectal temperatures) and circulatory parameters were unaffected by the experimental treatments. It should be remembered, however, that these men experienced little change in body K^+ despite efforts to alter K^+ storage.

CONCLUSION

In summary, these studies demonstrate the body's capacity to minimize electrolyte losses during acute and repeated bouts of exercise and dehydration. Although there are marked shifts in water and selected ions in the exercising muscle, only during prolonged exertion is the ratio of intra- to extramuscular K^+ significantly altered, which suggests that some modifications of the muscle cell membrane may occur. Muscle tissue not engaged in the exercise seems unaffected by the sweat lost during prolonged activity, but relinquishes intracellular water shortly after work is terminated. Blood, muscle, sweat, and urine measurements before and following varied levels of dehydration demonstrate that body water lost during exercise in the heat is accomplished at the expense of larger water losses from extracellular than from intracellular compartments. Moreover, the loss of ions in sweat and urine had little effect on the K^+ content of either plasma or muscle.

With repeated days of dehydration and heavy exercise, plasma volume increased in proportion to an increase in body Na^+ storage. At this point some mention should be made concerning the effect of this increased plasma water on the concentration of blood constituents. Because red blood cells and hemoglobin are confined to the vascular space, both may decrease significantly as a function of the hemodilution induced by repeated days of exercise and dehydration. This may in part explain the apparent anemia reported by sports physicians among athletes undergoing intensive training. It is also possible that such hemodilution may produce low concentrations of plasma K^+, which might be falsely interpreted as suggestive of a hypokalemic state. In any event, some caution should be used in the clinical interpretation of plasma concentrations of various constituents among endurance trained athletes.

With regard to the question of possible body K^+ depletion during repeated days of heavy exercise, calculations of K^+ balance (intake minus excretion) and measurements of plasma and muscle K^+ content fail to confirm the large deficits previously reported by Knochel, Dotin, and Hamburger (1972). Despite low dietary K^+ intake, little change in total body K^+ (<2% change) was observed, and there was an increase in muscle K^+ content. In the presence of a low K^+ intake there were strong suggestions that the kidneys were selectively conserving K^+. Future studies are needed to confirm this response, and to provide some explanation for the apparent increase in muscle K^+ content.

REFERENCES

Åstrand, P.-O, and Saltin, B. 1964. Plasma and red cell volume after prolonged severe exercise. J. Appl. Physiol. 19: 829–832.

Bartter, F. C., and Gann, D. S. 1960. On the hemodynamic regulation of the secretion of aldosterone. Circulation 21: 1016–1021.

Bergström, J. 1962. Muscle electrolytes in man. Determination by neutron activation analysis on needle biopsy specimens. A study on normal subjects, kidney patients, and patients with chronic diarrhea. Scand. J. Clin. Lab. Invest. 18: 16–20.

Costill, D. L., Coté, R., and Fink, W. 1976. Muscle water and electrolytes following varied levels of dehydration in man. J. Appl. Physiol. 40(1): 6–11.

Costill, D. L., Coté, R., Miller, E., Miller, T., and Wynder, S. 1975. Water and electrolyte replacement during repeated days of work in the heat. Aviat. Space Environ. Med. 46(6): 795–800.

Costill, D. L., and Fink, W. J. 1974. Plasma volume changes following exercise and thermal dehydration. J. Appl. Physiol. 37: 521–525.

Costill, D. L., Kammer, W. F., and Fisher, A. 1970. Fluid ingestion during distance running. Arch. Environ. Health. 21: 520–525.

Costill, D. L., and B. Saltin. 1975. Muscle glycogen and electrolytes following exercise and thermal dehydration. In H. Howald (ed.), Biochemistry of Exercise II. University Park Press, Baltimore.

Costill, D. L., and Sparks, K. E. 1973. Rapid fluid replacement following thermal dehydration. J. Appl. Physiol. 34: 299–303.

Cunningham, J. N., Carter, N. W., Rector, F. C., and Seldin, D. W. 1971. Resting membrane potential difference of skeletal muscle in normal subjects and severely ill patients. J. Clin. Invest. 50: 49–59.

Dill, D. B., and Costill, D. L. 1974. Calculation of percentage changes in volumes of blood, plasma, and red cells in dehydration. J. Appl. Physiol. 37: 247–248.

Hartroft, P. M., and Hartroft, S. 1961. Regulation of aldosterone secretion. Brit. Med. J. 1: 1171–1179.

Hodgkin, A. L., and Horowicz, P. 1959. The influence of potassium and chloride ions on the membrane potential of single muscle fibers. J. Physiol. (London) 148: 127–160.

Johns, R. J. 1960. Microelectrode studies of muscle membrane potential in man. Neurol. Disord. 38: 704–713.

Kjellmer, I. 1964. The effect of exercise on the vascular bed of skeletal muscle. Acta Physiol. Scand. 62: 18–30.

Knochel, J. P., Dotin, L. N., and Hamburger, R. J. 1972. Pathophysiology of intense physical conditioning in a hot climate. I. Mechanisms of potassium depletion. J. Clin. Invest. 51: 242–255.
Kozlowski, S., and Saltin, B. 1964. Effect of sweat loss on body fluids. J. Appl. Physiol. 19: 1119–1124.
Mellander, S., Johansson, B., Gray, S., Jonsson, O., Lundvall, J., and Ljung, B. 1967. The effects of hyperosmolarity on intact and isolated vascular smooth muscle. Possible role in exercise hyperemia. Angiologica. 4: 310–322.
Miller, H. C., and Darrow, D. C. 1941. Relation of serum and muscle electrolytes, particularly potassium to voluntary exercise. Am. J. Physiol. 132: 801–807.
Rose, K. D. 1975. Warning for millions: Intense exercise can deplete potassium. Physician Sports Med. 3: 26–29.
Saltin, B. 1964a. Aerobic work capacity and circulation at exercise in man with special reference to the effect of prolonged exercise and/or heat exposure. Acta Physiol. Scand. Suppl. 230.
Saltin, B. 1964b. Circulatory responses to submaximal and maximal exercise after thermal dehydration. J. Appl. Physiol. 19: 1125–1132.
Schamadan, J. L., and Snively, W. D., Jr. 1967. Potassium depletion as a possible cause for heat stroke. Ind. Med. Surg. 36: 785–788.
Vellar, O. D. 1968. Studies on sweat losses of nutrients. I. Iron content of whole body sweat and its association with other sweat constituents, serum iron levels, hematological indices, body surface area and sweat rate. Scand. J. Clin. Lab. Invest. 21: 157–167.

Nutrition and Sport

Some Aspects of Athlete's Nutrition

V. A. Rogozkin

Modern society has contributed substantially to improving the attitude of people toward the problems of nutrition. The continuously increasing intensity of various aspects of human activity, the possibility of covering great distance in comparatively short time, and the constantly occurring changes in the natural food resources have all influenced the revision of concepts in nutrition sciences. At present, nutrition and food are considered to be by experts not only a necessity for supporting life but also an important factor in the regulation of various parameters of metabolism. Nutrition of sportsmen, like that of every other person, is aimed mainly at providing the organism with an adequate quantity of energy, plastic materials, and essential nutrients. Correctly organized nutrition for sportsmen during periods of intense physical and neuro-psychological loads increases their working capacity and creates the foundation for achieving high levels of physical performance.

Several basic principles apply to the rational organization of the nutrition of athletes. They are derived from experimental results of the effects of different physical loads on the metabolism of sportsmen. The main principles for creation of nutritional plans for athletes are considered separately here, and are as follows:

1. Providing the sportsman with necessary quantities of energy according to the energy expended during physical activity (Pokrovsky, 1976).
2. Adhering to the principles of balanced nutrition with reference to definite kinds of sport and the intensity of physical loads. This means providing for distribution of the calories in the ration with reference to the main alimentary components (proteins, lipids, and carbohydrates), and the balance between the main nutrients, vitamins, and microelements (Pokrovsky, 1975).
3. Choosing adequate forms of nutrition (food products, nutrients,

and their combinations) and numbers of feeding (3−6) during the time of intensive training, and precompetition and competition periods (Litvinova et al., 1976).

4. The use of alimentary factors for rapid weight reduction to bring the sportsman to a specific body weight.

5. The application of the principles of individualized nutrition based on the anthropometric, physiological, and metabolic characteristics of the sportsman and the state of his digestive organs, tastes, and habits.

PROVIDING NECESSARY QUANTITIES OF ENERGY

The first principle is linked to both the energy expenditure during sports exercises and its compensation at the expense of feeding. The size of energy expenditure varies extremely and depends not only on the kind of sport but also on the volume of the performed work. Energy expenditure may also vary substantially for the same kind of sport depending on the period of precontest preparation and the period during the match (Åstrand and Rodahl, 1970; Edington and Edgerton, 1976), and, of course, on the athlete's body weight. In modern sport, the principal factors determining the increase in the energy cost of training are the increases in training intensity and number of training sessions per week. In general, top level athletes participate in two or three practice sessions each day, which requires a modification in nutrition and dietary habits. It is recognized that only very limited estimations of the energy expenditures of sportsmen under these conditions are presently available. Accurate values of energy expenditures are lacking for athletes participating in 2−3 training sessions a day in different sports. This can be observed in the great variation in values reported by researchers from different countries. The values of energy expenditures in male volleyball players (body weight 70kg) from four different countries in 1975 are given as examples: In the Soviet Union, 4,500−5,500 kcal; German Democratic Republic, 4,500−5,500 kcal; Bulgaria, 4,200−4,600 kcal; Japan, 3,150−3,850 kcal. Another example can be seen in judo wrestling. In this sport the values of energy expenditures are as follows: Soviet Union, 4,500−5,500 kcal; Bulgaria, 4,200−4,800 kcal; Japan, 3,800−4,500 kcal. It is still difficult to say something definite about the real cause of such sharp variations. It is clear that reliable data are needed pertaining to the energy expenditures of top-class athletes performing in 2−3 training sessions each day. This is the basis on which all rational nutrition of future athletes must be built. Without knowing the values of energy expenditures for the modern training process, it is impossible to establish effective nutrition and dietary programs for these athletes.

BALANCED NUTRITION WITH
REFERENCE TO SPORT AND INTENSITY

The second principle provides for both the optimal distribution in the ration of the main nutritional compounds (proteins, lipids, and carbohydrates) and the retention of the essential balance in nutrients (vitamins and microelements) (Pokrovsky, 1976). Conceptualization of the concrete recommendations must be grounded on the latest theoretical and experimental data. For instance, there exists an opinion in sport that weight lifters need nutrition with much higher protein content than representatives of other speed-strength kinds of sport. However, in the experiments on weight lifters an inverse proportion was found between the protein content in the ration and its assimilation for a certain quantity of protein. Table 1 presents values that characterize the requirement of sportsmen for energy and the principal nutrients. The larger the energy expenditures, the higher the need for energy and principal nutrients, respectively. However, an excessive amount of protein content in the ration may cause an unfavorable effect on the man's body. In this connection the protein share of the total calories decreases slightly as the energy expenditure increases, i.e., 13% for the caloric ration of 4,500−5,000 kcal; 12% for 5,500−6,500 kcal; and 11% at

Table 1. The requirement for principal nutrients and energy for male sportsmen

Kind of sport	Energy expenditures (kcal)	Proteins (g)	Lipids (g)	Carbohydrates (g)
Chess, draughts	2,800−3,200	96−109	90−103	382−438
Acrobatics, gymnastics, track and field athletics, weight-lifting, fencing	3,500−4,500	120−154	113−145	478−615
Wrestling, swimming, sport games	4,500−5,500	154−174	145−177	615−765
Bicycle racing; ski racing, marathon	5,500−6,500	174−190	177−210	765−920

about 8,000 kcal. It is generally agreed that the optimal provision of protein can be achieved with an animal/vegetable ratio of 1.0.

ADEQUATE NUTRITION

The third principle requires that adequate forms of nutrition (foodstuffs, nutrients, and their combinations) be selected to meet the nutritional needs of the athlete. The set of foodstuffs included in the athlete's ration determines significantly the rate of their assimilation, and consequently affects the working capacity of the athlete. Careful attention must be paid to the role of special products of high biological value in the composition of the ration. A contrary opinion exists among Bulgarian experts, who believe that the nutrition of athletes should not be based merely upon the kind of sport but rather on the intensity of physical loads encountered in the sport. For instance, at exercises comprising maximal and submaximal physical loads, which are usually performed under conditions of significant anaerobic oxidations, they recommend the following ration: proteins, $2-2.2$ g/kg body weight; lipids, $1-5$ g/kg body weight; and carbohydrates, up to 10 g/kg body weight, with supplements of vitamin C and of the Vitamin B, B_1, B_2, B_6, and B_{12} groups.

ALIMENTARY FACTORS AND INDIVIDUALIZED NUTRITION

A few sports such as wrestling, boxing, and weight lifting have special nutritional requirements. Considerable experience has been gained in the role of nutrition in the rapid loss of body weight by athletes in these sports.

Individualized nutrition programs for sportsmen require an understanding of their habits, tastes, and other peculiarities. For example, an important factor is the rate of food passage through the digestive tract. There are data that indicate the rate of food passage in weight lifters to be two to three times as high as in normal healthy males, and that a high percentage of nitrogen assimilation occurs under these conditions.

CONCLUSION

Research dealing with the nutrition of athletes must concentrate on the problems associated with the demands for high level performance and maintenance of good health under the physical stress of one, two, or three training sessions per day. Investigations under both laboratory and natural conditions must be carried out to solve the following problems:

1. The effects of two and three daily training sessions on the principal functions of the organism
2. The mechanisms of adaptive shifts in the main organs and systems of the athlete
3. Evaluation of the role of both the feeding timetable and different nutrients in the maintenance of a high working capacity in sportsmen
4. Elaboration of special feeding regimens, sets of nutrients, and diets for optimum recovery of the organisms of sportsmen following periods of strenuous exercise

The solution of these problems will facilitate the scientifically-substantiated medical planning necessary for the development and maintenance of high working capacity in sportsmen. Meanwhile, the results of new research will serve as a source of additional information, which is necessary for the establishment of firm conclusions.

REFERENCES

Åstrand, P. O., and Rodahl, K. 1970. Textbook of Work Physiology, pp. 455–457. Pergamon Press, New Jersey.

Edington, D. W., and Edgerton, V. R. 1976. The Biology of Physical Activity. Houghton Mifflin Co., Boston.

Laricheva, K. A., Yalovaya, N. I., Smirnov, P. V., Shubin, V. I., Azizbekyan, G. A., Levachev, M. M., Belyayev, V. S., Kim, M. D., Saksonov, N. N., and Shamarina, T. M. 1976. Izuchenie potrebnostej organizma sportsmena w energii i osnownich pischewych weschestwach. (Study of athlete organism needs in energy and main food substances.) Nutr. Sport. 60–66.

Litvinova, V. N., Morozov, V. I., Pshendin, A. I., Fedorova, G. P., Feldkoren, B. I., Tshajkovski, V. C., and Rogozkin, V. A. 1976. Wlianie kratnosti pitania na obmen belkow w skeletnich mischzach i pecheni belich kris. (Effects of number of meals on the protein metabolism in skeletal muscles and liver in albino rats.) Vopr. Pitan. 4: 36–41.

Pokrovsky, A. A. 1975. Role Biochimii w Razwitii Nauki o Pitanii. (Role of Biochemistry in the Development of Nutrition Science.) Nauka, Moscow.

Pokrovsky, A. A. 1976. Nekotorie prinzipi postroenia razionalnogo pitania sportsmenow. (Some principles of athletes rational nutrition.) Nutr. Sport 4–12.

Rogozkin, V. A. 1976. Wozmoznie puti sozdania i ispolzowania produrtow dla pitania sportsmenow. (Possible ways of food products development and their application for nutrition of athletes.) Nutr. Sport 121–127.

Slonchev, P. V., and Afar, I. M. 1976. Problemi differenzirowannogo pitania w sporte. (Problems of differentiated nutrition in sport.) Nutr. Sport 23–27.

Study of Energy Metabolism and Nutritional Status of Young Athletes

I. I. Alexandrov, N. N. Shishina

Intensification of training in contemporary sport indicates the urgent need for special studies of the energy metabolism and adequate nutrition of athletes. These problems are of particular importance in children and youth because at this stage the complex processes of growth and formation of the organism of young athletes are combined with the systematic influence of intensive training. Such studies and basic data for dietary allowances for young athletes are still rare (Borisov, 1966; Mahkamov et al., 1971; Romanchenko, 1971).

Because of the lack of experimental data on energy metabolism of young athletes, the caloric values of their food rations have been determined according to allowances elaborated for ordinary school children by the USSR Nutrition Institute of the Academy of Medical Sciences (Slonim, 1954). It is about 2,400–2,800 kcal /24 hr for the age group 14–17 years.

According to some studies on the energy metabolism of boarding school pupils, the energy expenditures amount to 2,874–3,424 kcal /24 hr. On days when these pupils participated in physical education lessons, their energy expenditures reached up to 3,700 kcal (Kopteva, 1961; Borisov, 1965). One may assume that energy costs of the activities in sports boarding schools will be even higher. Therefore, a study was conducted on 115 pupils in the Leningrad Sports Boarding School during a period of extensive training. The energy metabolism and caloric values of the diet provided for the pupils were investigated.

Energy cost of activities were determined in groups of runners (seven boys with a mean age of 17.4 ± 0.8 years, a mean body weight of 66.9 ± 5.9 kg, and a mean height of 179.1 ± 7.0 cm), skiers (seven boys with a mean age of 15.9 ± 1.1 years, a mean body weight of 66.3 ± 7.5 kg, and a mean height of 172.9 ± 6.3 cm), and swimmers (eight boys with a mean age of 14.0 ± 0.2 years, a mean body weight of 58.5 ± 5.6 kg, and a mean height of 169.4 ± 6.5 cm). Gas analyses were performed on the "Spirolyt" -Junkalor Dessau (German Democratic Republic). Heart rate was recorded with a radio telemetric system, "Sport." The measurements were performed at rest, during an increasing work load (Anderson et al., 1971), and in the field setting of real sport training. The data on O_2 consumption and heart rate at different levels of work load were correlated for each subject. The heart rates recorded during training sessions were later used to determine energy expenditures by the well-known methods of time recording of the main activities (Vinogradov, 1969; Sherrer, 1967). The caloric intakes of athletes were analyzed using food composition tables (Pokrovsky, 1964). To evaluate the protein metabolism in 115 young athletes specialized in running, swimming, gymnastics, and skiing (two age groups of 11–13 and 14–17 years, males and females) total proteins in the blood were determined (Lowry et al., 1951) as well as protein fractions (Gurvich, 1955), hemoglobin (Predtechensky, 1964), and urea (Ceriotti and Spandrio, 1963). The amounts of vitamins B_1, B_2, and C in urine were also ascertained (Pokrovsky, 1969). In the morning the pupils were examined under basal conditions.

The basal metabolism rate (BMR) was as a rule 3–9% lower than the expected level, with nonsignificant differences (Table 1). The observed lower level of basal metabolism is evidently within the normal range, as reported by other workers (Marshak, 1946; Davidanova, 1949; Yakovlev, 1967). Fluctuations of basal metabolism within ± 25% in subjects enrolled in sport training were also observed. The comparison of basal metabolism with actual training loan on individual days during the week showed that the change of volume and intensity of training loads caused corresponding changes of the basal metabolic rate. These average values of metabolism at rest were used to determine the minimal 24-hr energy requirement of young athletes (Table

Table 1. Energy metabolism in young athletes at rest conditions

| Sports group | Main energy costs (M ± 6)[a] | | Excess of expected observed (%) | Minimum energy level (kcal/24 hr) |
	expected (kcal/min)	observed (kcal/min)		
Runners	1.279 ± 0.073	1.173 ± 0.107	9	1,687 ± 155
Skiers	1.294 ± 0.078	1.210 ± 0.163	7	1,738 ± 238
Swimmers	1.245 ± 0.082	1.212 ± 0.191	3	1,745 ± 274

[a] $p < 0.05$.

Table 2.   Specific energy expenditure during sports activity

Sports group	Duration of training (min)	Energy expenditure (kcal/min)	Heart rate (beats/min)	Mean level of consumption (in % of max O_2 consumption)	Energy expenditure during training (kcal)
Runners	70 ± 22	12.0 ± 2.5	147 ± 14	63	865 ± 195
Skiers	91 ± 17	12.9 ± 2.4	160 ± 12	70	1,176 ± 256
Swimmers	182 ± 2	7.0 ± 1.9	121 ± 10	46	1,277 ± 346

1), which does not differ significantly from the expected value of 1,800 kcal/24 hr (Lehmann, 1958).

The total duration of training loads of subjects was from 70 to 182 min per day. The highest energy expenditure and heart rates were found in skiers with an oxygen consumption of 70% of maximum. Somewhat lower values were found in runners with an oxygen consumption reaching 63% of the maximum. In swimmers the per minute values were lowest. The total energy expenditure caused by sports training was highest in swimmers. Close to them was the energy output in skiers, and the lowest energy expenditure during total training was recorded in runners (Table 2).

Analysis of results over 24-hr periods showed that energy expenditure was about the same for runners, swimmers, and skiers (Table 3). Some differences were found in the energy output related to body weight. For example, the highest energy expenditure was found in swimmers and somewhat lower levels in athletes participating in other sport disciplines (Table 3).

The ratio of energy cost of sports training to total energy output per 24 hr is remarkable. During relatively short periods of time (70–182 min) they spend from 25 to 36% of the total energy output per 24 hr.

The diets of young athletes showed the energy value of food ingested on the level of 3,889 ± 57 kcal/24 hr. In addition, the total serum proteins were within the physiological range (Table 4). Protein fractions also corresponded to the level ascertained in untrained healthy subjects (Kopteva, 1961). The average total protein values were not

Table 3.   Energy expenditure of pupils from sports boarding schools

Sports group	Total energy expenditure over 24 hr (M + 6)	
	(kcal)	(kcal/kg)
Runners	3,464 ± 202	52.3 ± 4.0
Skiers	3,619 ± 475	54.8 ± 6.0
Swimmers	3,558 ± 468	61.3 ± 8.8

Table 4. Indicators of protein metabolism in pupils from sports boarding school

| Subjects | | Total serum proteins (g/100 liters) | Albumin (%) | Globulins (%) | | | | | Albumin: globulin ratio | Urea (mg/100 ml) | Hb (g/100 liters) |
Age (years)	Sex			α_1	α_2	β	γ	Total			
11–13	Boys	8.2 ± 0.3	66.1 ± 2.0	4.7 ± 0.8	6.1 ± 0.6	8.1 ± 0.6	15.2 ± 1.3	34.1	1.9	22.6 ± 1.0	13.1 ± 0.1
	Girls	6.9 ± 0.2	65.9 ± 1.0	4.6 ± 0.5	5.6 ± 0.4	7.7 ± 0.6	17.2 ± 1.4	35.3	1.9	27.6 ± 1.9	13.1 ± 0.1
14–17	Boys	7.1 ± 0.2	67.5 ± 1.7	3.9 ± 0.7	5.1 ± 1.2	8.1 ± 0.5	15.3 ± 1.1	32.4	2.0	22.5 ± 2.0	14.1 ± 0.2
	Girls	7.3 ± 0.4	65.6 ± 1.7	4.6 ± 0.5	6.0 ± 0.4	8.1 ± 0.5	15.7 ± 0.8	34.4	1.9	30.3 ± 1.4	13.4 ± 0.2

Table 5.   Urinary vitamin excretion in pupils of sports boarding schools

Age (years)	Sex	Vitamin B_1 (μg/hr)	Vitamin B_2 (μg/hr)	Vitamin C (mg/hr)
11−13	Boys	38.9 ± 4.3	20.7 ± 1.6	0.16 ± 0.02
	Girls	16.9 ± 1.0	23.7 ± 3.0	0.23 ± 0.03
14−17	Boys	21.1 ± 4.0	24.5 ± 2.1	0.22 ± 0.02
	Girls	15.9 ± 1.6	24.0 ± 3.1	0.24 ± 0.03

Subjects (spanning Age/Sex columns)

found to depend on age, sex, or sports discipline. No significant deviations from the normal range were found in blood urea and hemoglobin (Table 4).

As can be seen in Table 5, the existing rations meet the requirements of young athletes with regard to vitamins B_1 and B_2, which was substantiated by urinary excretion analysis. The level of vitamin C, however, was insufficient.

The level of energy expenditure of pupils of sport schools depends mostly on their sport specialization. For instance, if the energy expenditure per kg body weight in skiers and runners was 51−54 kcal/24 hr, these parameters in swimmers were significantly higher, 61.5 kcal /24 hr. The latter observation could be ascribed to the fact that swimmers were engaged in training with total duration of 3 hr daily (two training sessions a day), whereas skiers and runners had just one training session a day with a total duration of up to 1.5 hr.

Another urgent question is to what extent the energy expenditure of young athletes is compensated for by their diet. It was ascertained that the caloric value of their rations was about 3,900 kcal /24 hr. Considering that the caloric value of food ingested should exceed the energy expenditure by 10−13% (Zimkin et al., 1955), one can assume that in general the rations described above met the energy needs of the pupils, and might serve as approximate norms for the young athletes of corresponding training and morphological characteristics.

The main principle of rational nutrition is not only an adequate caloric value of the diet necessary to meet energy expenditure, but also the balance of the most important nutrients (proteins, fats, carbohydrates, vitamins and mineral salts, etc.). The analysis from this aspect indicated the desirability of some improvement in the subjects. Specifically, a higher consumption of vegetables and fruits, and also a slight increase in the consumption of vegetable fats and a wider variety of available food products, would have improved the nutritional program.

REFERENCES

Anderson, K. L., Shephard, R. J., Denolin, H., Varnauskas, E., and Masironi, R. 1971. Fundamentals of Exercise Testing. World Health Organization, Geneva.

Borisov, A. P. 1961. Opredelenie energeticheskikh zatrat uchaschikhsia v shkolah-internatakh. (Determination of energy costs of boarding school pupils.) Vopr. Pytan. 1: 21−24. Moscow.

Borisov, A. P. 1965. Energeticheskie zatrati uchaschiksia 9−10 klassov shkol-internatov. (Energy costs of 9−10 graders in boarding schools.) Gig. Sanit. 10: 111−113. Moscow.

Borisov, A. P. 1966. Energeticheskie zatrati uchaschikhsia 7−8 klassov shkol-internatov. (Energy costs of 7−8 graders in boarding schools.) Vopr. Pytan. 5: 55−58. Moscow.

Ceriotti, G., and Spandrio, L. 1963. A spectrophotometric method for determination of urea. Clin. Chim. Acta 8: 295−299.

Daridanova, A. V. 1949. Osnovnoy obmen u sportsmenov v processe trenirovky. (Base metabolism in athletes in the process of training.) Dissertation, The Leningrad State Institute of Physical Culture, named after P.F. Lesgaft, Leningrad.

Gurvich, A. E. 1955. Isuchenie sivorotochnikh belkov metodom elektrophoresa na philtrovalnoi bumage. (The study of serum proteins by electrophorese using the filter paper.) Lab. Delo. 3: 3−9. Moscow.

Kopteva, I. A. 1961. Belkovie frakzii sivorotki krovi zdorovikh ludei. (Protein fractions of blood serum in healthy human subjects.) Proc. Kujbyshevsky Med. Inst. 17: 212−214. Kujbyshev.

Lehmann, G. 1958. Physiological basis of tractor design. Ergonomics 1: 197−206.

Lowry, O. H., Rosenbroygh, N. J., Farr, A. L., and Randall, R. J. 1951. Protein measurement with the Folin phenol reagent. J. Biol. Chem. 193: 265−275.

Mahkamov, G. M., Romanchenko, N. L., Shamunamedov, S. S., and Shakhov, A. Y. 1971. Osnovnye ukazaniya po organizacyi pitaniya vospitannikov sportivnyh shkol-internatov. (The principal instructions in organization of nutrition of pupils of sports boarding schools.) The Tashkent State Medical Institute Publishers, Tashkent.

Marshak, M. E. 1946. Fiziologya Cheloveka. (Physiology of Man.) Physical Culture and Sport Publishers, Moscow.

Pokrovsky, A. A. 1964. Rukovodstvo po Izucheniyu Pitaniya i Zdorovya Naseleniya. (Manual for the Study of Nutritional Status in Healthy Populations.) Medicina Publishers, Moscow.

Pokrovsky, A. A. 1969. Biokhimimcheskye Metody Issledovaniya v Klinike, pp. 469−484. (Biochemical Methods of Study in Clinics.) Medicina Publishers, Moscow.

Predtechensky, V. E. 1964. Rukovodstvo po Klinicheskim Laboratornim Issledovaniyam, pp. 15−18. (Manual for the Clinical Laboratory Studies.) Medicina Publishers, Moscow.

Romanchenko, N. L. 1971. Kobosnovaniyu norm belkovogo i vitaminnogo (B_2, PP i C) pitaniya detey i podrostkov sportsmenov. (Elaboration of norms of protein and vitamin (B_2, PP, C) nutrition of young athletes.) Dissertation, The Tashkent State Medical Institute, Tashkent.

Scherrer, G. 1967. Physiologie du Travail (Ergonomie). (Physiology of Work—Ergonomics.) Masson et Cie Editeurs, Paris.

Slonim, A. D. 1954. Obmen energiy v organizme. (Energy metabolism in the organism.) In K.M. Bikov (ed.), Utchebnik Fiziologiy. (The Handbook of Physiology.) Physical Culture and Sport Publishers, Moscow.

Yakovlev, N. N. 1967. Pitaniye Sportsmenovo (Athletes' Nutrition.) Physical Culture and Sport Publishers, Moscow.

Yeremenko, N. P. 1959. Izmeneniya osnovnogo obmena u sportsmenov pri trenirovke razlichnoi napravlennosti. (The change in the basic metabolism of athletes after different types of training.) Ukrain. Biokhimich. J. 31(1): 89–98. Kiev.

Vinogradov, M. I. 1969. Rukovodstvo po Fiziologiy Truda. (Physiology of Work Manual.) Medicine Publishers, Moscow.

Zimkin, N. V., Korobkov, A. V., Lehtman, Y. I., Egolinsky, Y. A., and Yarocky, A. I. 1955. Fisiologicheskiye Osnovy Fizicheskoy Kultury i Sporta. (Physiological Bases of Physical Culture and Sport.) Physical Culture and Sport Publishers, Moscow.

Food Intake, Energy Expenditure, and Nutrient Requirements of Polish Students of Physical Education

I. Celejowa, L. Namystowski, J. Wykurz

For many years in Poland, food allowances for academic canteens have been obligatory (Celczyńska and Wolf, 1970). At present, the same allowances are applied in the canteens for students of the Polish academic schools of physical education.

Investigations designed to develop food allowances for students of physical education in Poland were performed during two periods at the Laboratory of Athlete Nutrition, Department of Hygiene, Academy of Physical Education in Warsaw, as well as at other Polish academic schools.

FIRST PERIOD OF STUDY

The quantitative and qualitative aspects of the food intake as well as the energy expenditure of students living at the Students' Home of the Academy of Physical Education in Warsaw were investigated in 1961, 1962, 1963, and 1968 (Namystowski and Celejowa, 1962; Namystowski, 1964, 1965). Table 1 shows the nutritive value of the canteen food ration in those years.

The caloric value of the total food ingested by the female and male students increased to a mean value of 5,100 kcal over 7 years (Table 2). To verify whether such a high food intake was justified by the real requirements, 24-hr energy expenditures were determined twice: in 1963 (Namystowski, 1964) and in 1968 (unpublished data). The approximate evaluation in 1963 showed that the 24-hr mean energy expenditures amounted to about 4,600 kcal, and the caloric requirement was 5,100 kcal. However, it is known that the time spent on practical sport activities never coincides 100% with the planned time, as emphasized

Table 1.   Mean nutritive value of the gross food ration supplied in the canteen of the Academy of Physical Education in Warsaw in 1961, 1962, and 1968[a]

Observation period	Content of nutrients				
	Caloric value (kcal)	Total protein (g)	Fat (g)	Carbohydrates (g)	Vitamin C (mg)
June, 1961	3,719	94	110	598	111
October, 1961	3,567	82	112	574	86
April, 1962	4,024	103	84	694	92
May, 1963	3,633	87	99	566	96
November-December, 1968	3,880	107	116	601	159
Mean	3,765	95	104	607	109

[a] Namystowski and Celejowa (1962), Namystowski (1964, 1965).

by Durnin and Passmore (1969). Thus in 1968, in fourth-year female and male students, strict timing of all activities during the day was carried out (unpublished data). It was found that at the Academy of Physical Education, the practical sport activities are interrupted by breaks (standing, sitting, etc.) lasting from 33% (sport games) to 73% (track and field) of their total duration. Thus, in these studies the energy expenditure proved to be much lower than that tentatively calculated in 1963 (Namystowski, 1964), and it represented only 18% of the 24-hr energy expenditure (refer to Table 6).

Moreover, determinations were made of the individual energy expenditures of the first, second, and fourth-year students who were competitors of the second and third sport class, and trained for short-distance races in track and field at the sport club, AZS-Warszawa, and lived at the Students' Home. The 24-hr energy expenditures of these

Table 2.   Real canteen food intake and total food intake in students of the Academy of Physical Education in Warsaw during 1961–1968.

Food intake	Mean caloric value (kcal)
Gross canteen food intake	3,765
Leftovers	276
Actual (net canteen food intake)	3,489~3,500
Supplementary food intake	1,600
Total food intake	5,089~5,100

students averaged 3,200 kcal. The energy expenditures during sport activities accounted for 31% of the 24-hr expenditures, and the mean caloric requirements of all investigated students amounted to 3,250 kcal.

Thus, the caloric requirement of students of the Academy of Physical Education exceeded the caloric allowances for students' canteens in Poland (Celeczyńska and Wolf, 1970), but it was consistent with the allowance of 3,200 kcal adopted by FAO (Rao, 1969) for a standard man weighing 65 kg.

Consequently, the food ration supplied at this time in the canteen of Students' Home of the Academy of Physical Education (3,500 kcal) covered the real food requirement of students. Thus, no supplementary food intake was necessary. A supplement was not needed for meeting the energy requirements, but it was considered necessary for certain nutrient deficiencies.

For instance, the protein intake was too low (Table 3). Because the caloric value of the athletes' food ration ought to exceed the protein requirements by at least 13%, or more, the protein requirement of physical education students with mean body weights of 68 kg amounted to 112 g/subject per day, i.e., to 1.6 g per 1 kg of body weight. The total protein intake averaged 132 g. This indicated that the supplementary protein intake compensated for, and even exceeded, the protein deficiency in the canteen food ration. However, because of the faulty composition of the supplementary food intake, the fat and carbohydrate intake and the caloric value of the diet greatly increased spontaneously. During the 1968–1969 academic year, the mean gain in body weight amounted in female and male students to 2.3 and 3 kg, respectively. According to Charzewski (1964), the adipose tissue increased by 28.8% in third-year students as compared with second-year students.

Because the intake of milk, dairy products, and fruits during this period of study was a little too low, the supplies of vitamins A and C were too low. The vitamin C deficiency in the diet was confirmed by the low ascorbic acid level in blood and urine of female students examined by Tukiendorf (1967). Studies performed in 1968 indicated a great improvement—the total vitamin C intake averaged 159 mg/subject per day (see Table 1). However, after subtracting 50% for cooking losses, this intake amounted to only 71 mg, whereas the vitamin C allowance for athletes is 100–150 mg. Likewise, the intakes of other vitamins and mineral substances were improved.

On the basis of the results obtained in years 1961–1968 for the food intake and energy expenditure of physical education students in Warsaw, tentative nutrient allowances for physical education students were accepted (Celejowa, 1971). These allowances were higher than

Table 3. Gross canteen protein intake in students of the Academy of Physical Education in Warsaw during 1961–1968 compared with the obligatory protein allowance for Polish students' canteens and with the actual protein requirements[a]

Protein intake						Obligatory protein allowance[b]	Percentage of allowance met	Actual protein requirement	Percentage of the requirement met
June 1961	October 1961	April 1962	May 1963	Nov.–Dec. 1968	Mean				
94	82	103	87	107	95	97	98	112	85

[a] Celczyńska and Wolf, 1970.
[b] Celejowa and Kubinyi, 1968.

Table 4. Nutrient allowances proposed by Celejowa[a] for the canteens of Polish physical education students as compared with the required allowances for Polish students[b]

Nutrient	Gross value		Net value after subtracting 10% for cooking losses	
	Required allowance	Allowance for physical education students	Required allowance	Allowance for physical education students
Calories (kcal)	3,450	3,750	3,110	3,407
Total protein (g)	97	122	87	112
Animal protein (g)	46	103	42	93
Fat (g)	110	118	100	107
Carbohydrates (g)	516	549	465	499
Calcium (g)	1.2	1.7	1.1	1.5
Iron (mg)	24	27	21	24
Vitamin A (IU)	1,410	4,533	1,280	4,120
Carotene converted to Vitamin A (IU)	10,570	14,562	9,500	13,238
Vitamin B_1 (mg)	2.2	3.0	2.0	2.7
Vitamin B_2 (mg)	2.1	2.8	1.8	2.5
Vitamin C (mg)	151	170	136	135

[a] Celejowa, 1971.
[b] Celczyńska and Wolf, 1970.

the allowances required for student canteens in all types of academic schools in Poland, as presented in Table 4 (Celczyńska and Wolf, 1970).

SECOND PERIOD OF STUDY

In recent years, the Polish academic schools of physical education have undergone great changes. At present the structure of the student population is quite different than that of the first period of this study. In the first period only 9.3% of the total student population were competitors, whereas at present the competitors comprise 36% of the students. Thus, it became necessary to repeat the studies and to bring the food allowances up to date. In 1972, studies were carried out in the canteen of Students' Home of the Academy of Physical Education in Warsaw (Celejowa and Wykurz, 1972). At the same time, the energy expenditures of first-year students who trained as competitors at the Sport Club were investigated in cooperation with the Medical Academy in Warsaw. These results are shown in Table 5 (Celejowa and Wykurz, 1972).

Table 5. Energy costs of some selected activities belonging to the curriculum of first-year students at the Academy of Physical Education[a]

Sex	N	Body weight (kg)	Body stature (cm)	Age (years)	Activity	Energy cost	
						kcal/min/kg	kcal/min
Male	6	66 ± 9.75	173.8 ± 10.51	19.7 ± 0.61	Games	0.075 ± 0.027	4.8 ± 1.51
	4	70.9 ± 7.44	176.7 ± 9.57	19.5 ± 0.57	Exercises with music	0.078 ± 0.013	5.6 ± 1.47
Female	4	75.8 ± 4.19	180.0 ± 4.96	19.0	Basketball	0.133 ± 0.074	9.9 ± 4.90
	4	61.0 ± 8.40	165.5 ± 2.08	19.5 ± 0.37	Exercises with music	0.072 ± 0.016	4.4 ± 1.28
	6	55.2 ± 8.86	161.8 ± 6.61	19.3 ± 0.51	Basketball	0.102 ± 0.042	5.4 ± 1.7
	4	61.8 ± 6.23	166.8 ± 4.11	19.7 ± 1.7	Games	0.057 ± 0.019	3.5 ± 1.15

[a] Celejowa and Wykurz (1972).

Table 6. Daily energy expenditure of Polish physical education students as compared with the world student population

Academic school and year of study	Mean energy expenditures (kcal, rounded to nearest hundred)
Academy of Physical Education, Warsaw,[a] 1968	3,000
Academy of Physical Education, Warsaw,[a] 1972	4,300
World student population[b]	2,600

[a] From dissertations of M.S. degree students under the direction of I. Celejowa.
[b] From Durnin and Passmore (1969) and Durnin (1970).

The mean daily energy expenditure of first-year students training as competitors within the sport activity program of the Academy of Physical Education in Warsaw was about 4,300 kcal (Table 6). By participating in sport activities, the students, on the average, increased their mean daily energy expenditures by 36% on an average of 1,200 kcal, as compared with the first period of studies. Therefore, at present the caloric requirements of students who are highly qualified competitors amount to 4,700 kcal/day per 70 kg, and are about 1,000 kcal higher than the allowances recommended in 1971 (Celejowa, 1971).

It is worthwhile to evaluate the nutritive value of the canteen food ration, which is consistent with the allowances still being required for all student canteens in Poland. The food ingested in the canteen of the Academy of Physical Education in Warsaw failed to meet the nutrient requirements of student competitors. The caloric value of this food ration was 3,423 kcal (Table 7), and it was 1,300 kcal (i.e., about 28%) lower than the students' real caloric requirement. Protein intake met 77% of the actual protein requirement, fat intake covered 62% of the fat requirements, and carbohydrate intake was 75% of the carbohydrate requirements (Table 8).

A similar nutrient requirement was found in physical education students during ski training camp for first-year students of the Academy of Physical Education in Warsaw in 1974, and in 1972 at the Academy of Physical Education in Cracow (Emmerich, Kubica, and Klimek, 1972) (Table 9). Thus, the mean daily energy expenditure of students training as competitors within the sport activities at the Academy of Physical Education or training at a ski camp was 4,225 kcal (Table 9), whereas, that of the students practicing sport only during ski training camps amounted to 4,200 kcal. Therefore, the caloric requirements (daily energy expenditure + 10%) of ski camp participants resembled that of the first-year students training as competitors

Table 7. Nutritive value of the gross food ration supplied in the canteen of the Academy of Physical Education in November, 1972, according to chemical analysis as compared with the allowances for Polish students' canteens and allowances for physical education students proposed in 1971

Nutrient	Canteen nutrient[d]	Allowance[a]	Percentage of allowance	Allowance[b]	Percentage of allowance	Mean in previous years
Calories (kcal n)	3,423	3,750	91	3,450	99	3,765
Total protein (g)	118	123	96	97	122	95
Fat (g)	91	118	77	110	83	104
Carbohydrates (g)	522	549	95	516	101	607

[a] Celejowa and Wykurz (1972).
[b] Celczyńska and Wolf (1970).
[c] Celejowa (1971).
[d] Charzewski (1964).

Table 8.   Comparison of the nutritive value of the food ration supplied in the canteen of the Academy of Physical Education in Warsaw[a] in 1972 with the actual requirements of student competitors

Nutrient	Canteen food ration	Actual requirement	Percentage of requirement met
Caloric value (kcal n)	3,423	4,700	72
Protein (g)	118	153	77
Fat (g)	91	146	62
Carbohydrates (g)	522	693	75

[a] Celejowa and Wykurz (1972).

within the sport activities at the Academy, which was 4,620 kcal (Table 10).

Students of the Academy of Physical Education in Warsaw not practicing sport as competitors accounted for 64% (including 39% women) of the total student population. Their nutrient requirements corresponded to the allowances estimated in 1971 at 3,750 kcal (Celejowa, 1971). Thus, at present the mean caloric requirement of the entire student population, consisting of both competitors and noncompetitors, with mean body weight of 69 kg is about 4,100 kcal.

Deficiencies in the nutritive value of the food ration supplied in the canteen of the Academy of Physical Education in Warsaw, according to the Cracow studies (Celejowa and Kubinyi, 1968) and in other Polish academic canteens as well, were compensated for by supplementary food intakes (Table 11).

Table 9.   Mean daily energy expenditure of Polish physical education students from 1972–1974

Academic school and year of study	Energy expenditure (kcal)
Academy of Physical Education, Warsaw, 1972[a]	4,300
Academy of Physical Education, Warsaw ski camp, 1974[a]	4,000
Academy of Physical Education, Cracow ski camp, 1972[b]	5,000 (male students) 3,600 (female students)
Mean	4,225

[a] From dissertations of M.S. degree students under the direction of I. Celejowa.
[b] From Emmerich, Kubica, and Klimek (1972).

Table 10.   Daily energy expenditure and mean caloric requirements of physical education students during ski training camps investigated in 1972 and 1974

Academic school and year of study	Daily energy expenditure (kcal)	Mean caloric requirement (mean daily energy + 10%)
Academy of Physical Education, Cracow, 1972	5,000 (male 3,600 (female)	
Academy of Physical Education, Warsaw, 1974	4,000 (male)	
Mean	4,200	4,620

[a] From Emmerich, Kubica, and Klimek (1972).
[b] From dissertations of M.S. degree students under the direction of I. Celejowa.

REVISED FOOD ALLOWANCES FOR PHYSICAL EDUCATION STUDENTS IN POLAND

On the basis of the previously mentioned investigations, and at the order of the Chief Committee of Physical Culture and Tourism, modified food allowances for physical education students in Poland were proposed (Table 12). In these revised allowances it was assumed that the student population is composed of 36% competitors (mean body weight 70 kg) and 64% noncompetitors (mean body weight 69 kg). The revised allowances represent the mean allowances for these two groups of students. Moreover, the allowances include the proposed mean food ration expressed in food products as well as the nutrient content of this food ration. Because the intensity of work of physical education students is variable, it was assumed that the food ration expressed in food

Table 11.   Total food intake of students of the Academy of Physical Education in Warsaw from 1972–1973 as compared with revised allowances[a]

Nutrient	Food intake			Allowance	Percentage of allowance met
	In canteen	Supplementary	Total		
Protein (g)	118.2	24.1	142.3	133	107
Fat (g)	90.8	37.7	128.5	128	100.7
Carbohydrates (g)	522.0	106.8	628.8	605	104.0
Calories (kcal)	3,423.4	871.5	4,294.9	4,100	104.9

[a] Proposed by Celejowa and Wykurz (1972).

Table 12a. Revised food allowances for Polish students of physical education[a]

Proposed daily food rations in food products[b]		
Number	Product	Amount (g)
1.	Cereals	400
	bakery products	412
	flour and alimentary pastes	45
	groats	40
2.	Milk and dairy products	1,100
	milk	500
	cottage cheese	35
3.	Eggs	1 egg
4.	Meat, sausages, and fish	410
	meat	240
	sausages	85
	fish	60
5.	Butter	40
	butter	35
	cream (20%)	30
6.	Other fats	30
7.	Potatoes	400
8.	Vegetables and fruits rich in vitamin C	310
	cabbage	90
	tomatoes	200
	fruits	20
9.	Vegetables rich in carotene	160
10.	Other vegetables and fruits	500
	vegetables	250
	fruits	190
	dried fruits	13
11.	Dry legumes	10
12.	Sugar	180
	sugar	135
	jams and marmalades	90

Weight ratio of protein:fat:carbohydrates—1:0.96:4.5
Weight ratio of animal protein:vegetable protein—1:0.3
Ratio of calcium:phosphate—1:1.5
Ratio of percentages of calories from protein:fat:carbohydrates—13:28:59

[a] Celejowa (1977).
[b] Calculated from tables for commercial products (Szczygieł et al., 1972).

Table 12b.   Revised food allowances for Polish students of physical education

| | Recommended nutrient allowances for this population group | | Content of nutrients in the proposed food ration | |
| | Allowance per: | | | |
Nutrient and unit	69 kg	1 kg	Raw	Cooked[a]
Calories (kcal n)	4,100	59.42	4,140	4,600
Total protein (g)	133	1.93	153	138
animal protein (g) (about three-fourths of total protein)	102		140	103
Fat (g)	128	1.85	126	
Carbohydrates (g)	605	8.77	608	686
Calcium (g)	1.0		1.5	1.7
Phosphorus (g)	1.5		2.2	2.5
Iron (mg)	12		27	30
Vitamin A (IU) (together with carotene converted to vitamin A)	6,600		14,100	15,670
Vitamin B_1 (mg)	2.2		2.5	2.8
Vitamin B_2	2.0		2.3	2.5
Vitamin C (mg)	112		203	225

[a] The cooked values take into account the cooking losses, estimated at 10%.

products must contain a fairly large safety margin, corresponding to the economic level C of balanced nutrition, as specified by Szczygieł, Siczkówna, and Nowicka (1970). The present allowances were established according to the method applied in this publication. However, lower levels of cereals, potatoes, and fats, as well as greater quantities of milk, meat, fruits, and sugar were proposed. This result stemmed from the need for taking into account the specific nature of athlete's nutrition, namely an increased requirement for protein, mineral components, and vitamins, and reduced requirements for fats, as well as higher energy requirements simultaneously with the maintenance of a small volume of food.

The food ration supplied, in compliance with these allowances, in canteens for physical education students may fail to fully meet the requirements of the part of the student population comprising highly qualified competitors, and it may be excessive for the other part of the student population (noncompetitors). These difficulties can be overcome by adjustments in the sizes of helpings as well as by continuation of the present system of supplying supplementary food to highly qualified competitors, as practiced at the Sport Club AZS.

Table 13a. Revised gross nutrient allowances recommended[a] for canteens for physical education students as compared with the required allowances for Polish student canteens

	Nutritive value	
Nutrient	Required allowance (gross)	Allowance[b]
Calories (kcal n)	3,450	4,600
Protein (g)	97	153
Fat (g)	110	140
Carbohydrates (g)	516	686
Calcium (g)	1.2	1.7
Iron (mg)	24	30
Vitamin A (IU) (together with carotene converted to vitamin A)	11,980	15,670
Vitamin B_1 (mg)	2.2	2.8
Vitamin B_2 (mg)	2.1	2.5
Vitamin C (mg)	151	225

[a] Celejowa (1977).
[b] The nutritive value is calculated for commercial products (Celejowa, 1977).

Table 13b. Revised gross nutrient allowances recommended for canteens for physical education students as compared with the required allowances for Polish student canteens

	Daily food ration expressed in food products		
Number	Product	Required allowance (g)	Allowance[a] (g)
1.	Cereals	400	400
2.	Milk and dairy products	875	1,100
3.	Eggs	0.5	1
4.	Meat, sausages, and fish	155	410
5.	Butter	28	40
6.	Other fat	32	30
7.	Potatoes	465	400
8, 9, 10.	Vegetables and fruits	640	970
11.	Dry legumes	12	10
12.	Sugar and sweets	68	180

[a] Celejowa (1977).

CONCLUSIONS

1. The food allowances required for all student canteens in Poland were, on the grounds of the performed studies, found to be too low for physical education students (Table 13).

2. Food allowances for Polish physical education students, developed on the basis of several years of study, amounted to: 4,100 kcal, 133 g protein, 128 g fat, and 605 g carbohydrates (calculated per mean body weight of 69 kg). When calculated per 1 kg of body weight, these allowances are: 59 kcal, 1.93 g protein, 1.85 g fat, and 8.77 g carbohydrates.

3. Studies of the energy expenditure and nutrient requirements of physical education students in Poland are continuing in order to modify, from time to time, the revised allowances with the changing conditions of life, work, and training.

REFERENCES

Celczyńska, J., and Wolf, K. 1970. Nutrition in students' canteens. Watra, Warsaw.

Celejowa, I. 1971. Kultura Fizyczna 8: 367–372.

Celejowa, I., and Kubinyi, A. 1968. Bull. Birsh Bureau Inf. Res. Stud. Health 5: 48.

Celejowa, I., and Wykurz, J. 1972. Nutrient requirement of 1st year students of the Academy of Physical Education, determined from their energy expenditure, as compared with the nutritive value of canteen food rations in November 1972. Submitted for publication.

Charzewski, J. 1964. Roczniki Naukowe AWF w Warszawie.

Durnin, J. V. G. A. 1970. Nutrition, pp. 321–323. Excerpta Medica, Amsterdam.

Durnin, J. V. G. A., and Passmore, R. 1969. Energy, work and leisure. Transl. by H. Kociuba and S. Kozłowski. PWN, Warsaw.

Emmerich, J., Kubica, R., and Klimek, A. 1972. Wychowanie Fizyczne i Sport 4: 79–85.

Namysłowski, L. 1964. Kultura Fizyczna 10: 608–617.

Namysłowski, L. 1965. Kultura Fizyczna 6: 334–344.

Namysłowski, L., and Celejowa, I. 1962. Kultura Fizyczna 5: 405–412.

Rao, K. K. P. N. 1969. Abstracts of Papers. In J. Mašek et al. (eds.), VIIIth International Congress of Nutrition, p. 562, August 28–September 5, Prague.

Szczygieł, A., Klimczak, Z., Piekarska, J., Muszkatowa, B. 1972. Tables of the composition and nutritive value of food products. PZWL, Warsaw.

Szczygieł, A., Siczkówna, J., Nowicka, L. 1970. Food allowances for eighteen population groups. PZWL, Warsaw.

Tukiendorf C. 1967. Kultura Fizyczna 7: 311–313.

Aims and Results of Dietary Surveys on Athletes

A. Ferro-Luzzi, A. Venerando

It is generally accepted that the evaluation of the nutritional status of individuals or populations can provide an objective standard for the assessment of the adequacy of dietary intakes. However, the available standards of reference for the evaluation of the nutritional status in relation to age, sex, and height seem to be inadequate when applied to athletes participating in different sport activities.

The nutritional status of the athletes may differ widely with respect to the ideal pattern of a healthy and adequately-nourished individual because of a number of factors related to the sport, to the anthropometric characteristics peculiar to and conditioning for the performance of a specific sport, and to the adaptive changes induced by training. The relation between the fat-free mass and the fat mass of the athletes, for example, can undergo remarkable variations, depending on the anthropometric characteristics required in specific sports, to achieve the best performance from a functional and biomechanical point of view.

As a very general rule, the ideal is represented by low ponderal index, low fat percentage, and relative muscular hypertrophy. However, there are certainly exceptions to this rough rule. Middle and long distance runners, for example, have a greater height and lesser weight on the average, and an evaluation of their nutritional status would classify them as undernourished and as having a delicate constitution.

Thus, a correct evaluation of the adequacy of the dietary intakes of athletes cannot be based on apparent nutritional status, at least until specific proper standards of reference are available for those sports in which explicit structural qualities necessary for the achievement of a satisfying performance are involved. Until then, an assessment of the dietary intakes would be the most precise and practical way to explore the nutritional equilibrium of an athlete, from the quantitative and qual-

Table 1.   Distribution of 406 athletes according to their physiological activity

Type of performance	Subjects N	Type of sport	Men	Women
Aerobic effort	61	Cross country skiing	20	
		Swimming	1	1
		Cycling (road events)	28	
		Walking	3	
		Marathon	1	
		Track and field (1,500m-5,000m-10,000 m)	5	2
Alternate aerobic and anaerobic effort	100	Volleyball	18	
		Basketball	16	
		Water polo	13	
		Boxing	43	
		Wrestling	5	
		Judo	5	
Massive aerobic-anaerobic effort	80	Skating	8	2
		Swimming (100m, 200m, all styles)	1	
		Canoeing (kayak)	59	5
		Track and field (400m hurdles, 400 and 800m)	3	2
Power activity	17	Weight lifting	5	
		Shot put		2
		Hammer	1	
		Javelin	1	
		100m-200m-110 hurdles, 100 hurdles	3	1
		High jump	1	
		Pole vault	2	
		Triple jump	1	
Skill activity	148	Bobsledding	43	
		Luge		3
		Riding	2	
		Yachting (all classes)	7	
		Gymnastics	15	13
		Fencing	13	5
		Alpine skiing	22	1
		Target shooting	24	

itative point of view. However limited by mistakes inherent in the method or by the lack of agreement on the optimal intake of nutrients for various sports, the surveys on food consumption are useful to ascertain possible deficiencies and/or partial or total excesses. Moreover, these surveys can provide indirect but valuable information on the energy cost of sport activities still largely missing.

A general criticism of dietary surveys is that the dietary intakes of the athlete may reflect imposed models of erroneous practices and food fads still largely present in the sports world rather than the real biological needs (Gounelle and Berard, 1966; Mickelsen, 1970; Cho and Freyer, 1974; S'Jongers, Dufaux, and Anseeuw, 1976).

Nevertheless, surveys conducted on spontaneous dietary intakes of athletes may be very useful for the progress of knowledge about the nutritional requirements of subjects such as athletes, whose nutritional status is fundamental for optimal performance. Such surveys may also provide useful information in regard to the range within which the human organism tolerates possible dietary mistakes without a detrimental effect on performance and the influence of an adequate diet on training and performance.

In spite of the importance attributed to a correct diet for the training and performing athlete, representative reliable documentation on what the athlete habitually and spontaneously eats is still largely missing.

A study conducted in 1972 on the diets of 425 Italian athletes who applied for participation in the 1972 Munich Olympic Games has provided some insight into this topic (Ferro-Luzzi, Topi, and Caldarone, 1975; Ferro-Luzzi, Caldarone, and Topi, 1976). This group was composed for the most part of men. The physical characteristics of the subjects and their distribution in various sport categories (Dal Monte, 1969) are shown in Tables 1 and 2.

Table 2.   Age and physical characteristics of the subjects

Sports group	Subjects N	Age (years) M	SD	Weight (kg) M	SD	Height (cm) M	SD
Men							
Aerobic	58	25.1	± 2.9	70.3	± 7.0	175.8	± 5.6
Aerobic-anaerobic alternate	100	22.8	± 3.1	74.5	± 14.2	176.1	± 13.8
Aerobic-anaerobic massive	71	23.2	± 3.3	79.7	± 9.6	181.2	± 13.9
Power	14	24.1	± 2.4	80.4	± 16.8	177.0	± 10.7
Skill with relevant muscular effort	52	22.5	± 3.7	68.4	± 6.4	172.9	± 6.0
Skill with little muscular effort	74	26.7	± 5.7	77.3	± 9.7	175.7	± 5.7
Women							
Aerobic-anaerobic massive and power	15	20.7	± 3.4	56.1	± 5.5	163.5	± 6.7
Skill with relevant muscular effort	22	18.5	± 5.8	53.3	± 22.0	160.3	± 6.7

The dietary intakes were assessed by an interview, during which the quantitative and qualitative aspects of the food consumption were investigated, with emphasis on the assessment of usual consumption. The validity of this procedure was increased by the rather high constancy in the custom of food usage of the athlete. The nutrient content of the diets was calculated with the aid of the Italian tables of food composition (INN, 1972).

The mean daily energy intake of the different groups of athletes is shown in Table 3. There were obvious differences among the groups. Group 1 had the highest daily energy intake, 4,337 kcal, and Group 5 the lowest, 3,358 kcal. The two female groups showed lesser energy intakes compared to the male athletes. When body weight was taken into consideration, energy intakes ranged from a minimum of 46 kcal/ kg body mass in Group 6 to a maximum of 62 kcal/kg body mass in Group 1. Female athletes had relatively high values, the girls of Group 3 having the second highest value of energy intake/kg body mass, independent of sex.

The daily total protein, fat, and carbohydrate intakes of the subjects are shown in Table 4. The intakes of the total protein represented one of the highest intakes ever recorded in Italy, reaching almost 200 g/day for Groups 1, 3, and 4. Expressed in terms of body mass, the protein intake was nearly 3 g/kg body mass for the males of Group 1

Table 3.   The mean daily energy intake of Italian athletes

Sport groups	Subjects N	Daily energy intake		
		kcal	SD	kcal / kg
Men				
1. Aerobic	58	4,337	± 1,146	62
2. Aerobic-anaerobic-alternate	100	3,751	± 731	50
3. Aerobic-anaerobic-massive	71	4,184	± 916	53
4. Power	14	4,150	± 818	52
5. Skill with relevant muscular effort	52	3,358	± 532	49
6. Skill with little musuclar effort	74	3,520	± 850	46
Women				
3. Aerobic-anaerobic-massive	15	3,211	± 701	57
5. Skill with relevant muscular effort	22	2,772	± 524	52

Table 4. Total mean daily nutrient intake of Italian athletes

Sport group	Subjects N	Total protein g	SD	g/kg	Fat g	SD	CHO g	SD
Men								
1. Aerobic	58	194	± 37	2.8	118	± 34	558	± 122
2. Aerobic-anaerobic- alternate	100	181	± 35	2.4	116	± 34	444	± 119
3. Aerobic-anaerobic- massive	71	195	± 48	2.5	130	± 40	498	± 154
4. Power	14	196	± 62	2.4	134	± 47	496	± 98
5. Skill with relevant muscular effort	52	168	± 32	2.5	110	± 25	393	± 92
6. Skill with little muscular effort	74	171	± 48	2.2	104	± 35	401	± 143
Women								
3. Aerobic-anaerobic- massive	15	160	± 30	2.9	109	± 24	374	± 146
5. Skill with relevant muscular effort	22	143	± 31	2.7	103	± 24	306	± 87

and the females of Group 3. On the other hand, the fat content of the diets was rather low, ranging between 104 and 135 g/day.

A general picture of what these subjects eat in terms of foods expressed as percentage of the total energy contributed by various food groups may be gained from Figure 1, where the contribution of the various food groups to total energy intake is presented. Over one-third of the total energy intake was derived from Italian staples such as bread, pasta, and rice. Next came milk and dairy products (13%). Meat (fresh and processed) contributed another 13% of the total energy intake. Only just over 1% was derived from eggs.

Visible fats (including all kinds of oil, margarine, and butter) provided about 11% of the total energy intake, which was relatively low and reflected the attitude of the Italian athlete toward fats. Sugar, jams, and sweets had a relevant position, contributing 9% of the total energy intake. Another 8% was derived from fresh vegetables, potatoes, and fruits. Alcohol contributed a low 5%, with a range of 3 to 7% within the various groups.

Compared to males, the female athletes derived a smaller percentage of the total energy from bread, pasta, and rice, and a comparably higher contribution from meat, milk and cheese, fruits, and vegetables.

In comparison with the average Italian diet (Table 5), the most important differences appeared in the consumption of bread, pasta, and rice, which contributed nearly 40% of the total energy of the diet of the

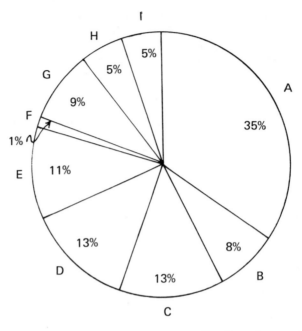

A — Bread, pasta, rice
B — Vegetables, potatoes, fruits
C — Meat, salami
D — Eggs
E — Milk, cheese
F — Miscellaneous

G — Sugar jams and
      sweet
H — Alcohol
I — Miscellaneous

Figure 1. Percentage of the total energy intake from food groups (athletes P.O. 1972).

average Italian, while these foods ranged between 27 and 37% for the athlete. Even more accentuated was the different contribution of salami and cheese: two to almost three times higher in the athletes. Comparison of the percentage of energy derived from butter, oil, and margarine showed a higher contribution from butter and a lower one from oil in the diet of the athletes. Alcohol contribution to total energy intake of the athletes, although variable, seemed to be lower on the average than the Italian value.

The contribution to protein intake from various food groups is shown in Figure 2. The values are the average of all groups of male athletes. Nearly half the total amount consumed was derived from meat; milk and cheese provided jointly 21% of the total protein intake, and eggs only 2%. Bread, pasta, and rice contributed some 23%. The consumption of fish was of such a minute amount that it might be considered negligible.

Table 5. Energy intake from foods and food groups (expressed as percent of total)

	Sport groups[a]							Italian average (ISTAT, 1971)
	Men						Women	
Foods	1	2	3	4	5	6	3 + 5	
Bread, pasta, rice	36	36	34	34	37	36	27	39
Vegetables[b]	2	2	2	2	2	2	3	4
Fruits[c]	6	6	5	6	6	5	7	4
Meat, Salami	13	12	13	12	14	15	16	6
Eggs	1	1	1	2	1	1	1	1
Milk	4	4	6	3	4	5	4	4
Cheese	5	10	10	11	10	9	11	3
Butter	4	2	2	3	2	2	3	1
Oil, margarine	8	9	8	9	9	8	8	15
Sugar	3	3	3	2	3	3	3	11
Jams[d]	6	7	7	3	8	6	10	
Alcohol	3	7	5	6	3	5	1	8
Miscellaneous	9	1	4	7	1	5	6	4

[a] 1, Aerobic; 2, Aerobic-anaerobic-alternate; 3, Aerobic-anaerobic-massive; 4, Power; 5, Skill with relevant muscular effort; 6, Skill with little muscular effort.

[b] Including potatoes.

[c] Fresh and canned.

[d] Including also marmalades, candies, and sweet beverages.

The percentage of total protein derived from various food groups has been compared in the six sport groups as well as with the average Italian values in Table 6. Some differences may be noticed, although it is difficult to interpret their meaning. It may be seen that the athletes of Group 1 obtained more protein from bread, pasta, and rice than did the athletes of the other groups. Athletes of Group 3 seemed to consume more milk and cheese and less meat. Women athletes relied more than men on meat; their bread, pasta, and rice consumption contributed significantly lower amounts to total protein intake. The differences between the average Italian dietary pattern and that of the athletes are shown in the last column of Table 6. The main difference was represented by a considerably lower contribution of meat and cheese to the total protein intake of the average Italian, and bread, pasta, rice, vegetables, eggs, and milk provided a higher percentage of their total protein intake. The results of this study show that the diet of the Italian athlete differs from the diet commonly consumed in Italy. The most important feature of these differences, without doubt, is the high protein intake and the prominent position of meat.

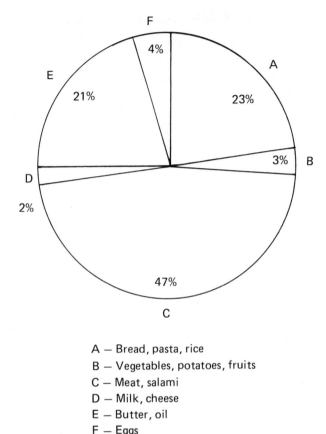

A — Bread, pasta, rice
B — Vegetables, potatoes, fruits
C — Meat, salami
D — Milk, cheese
E — Butter, oil
F — Eggs

Figure 2. Percentage of the total protein intake from foods and food groups (athletes P.O. 1972).

The diets consumed by these athletes may be considered "spontaneous" inasmuch as they were not obviously "on a diet," nor did they report that they followed specific dietary advice of any sort. However, it must be noted that this so-called "spontaneous" diet was probably the result of the interaction of at least two factors: the current Italian dietary pattern and the specific beliefs and "hearsays" of the world of sport.

We can, therefore, recognize, for example, in the low egg consumption of 26 g/day/person the role of the first series of factors. Average Italian consumption gives a very similar value of 32 g/day/person (ISTAT, 1971). The cause of these low figures may be a multitude of factors, including marketing, distribution, or cost of the commodity. However, the major cause of the limited consumption of eggs seems to be attributable to a negative attitude toward this food associated, in the

Table 6.   Protein intake from foods and food groups (expressed as percent of total)

| Foods | Sport groups[a] | | | | | | | Italian average (ISTAT, 1971) |
| | Men | | | | | | Women | |
	1	2	3	4	5	6	3+5	
Bread, pasta, rice	27	23	23	22	24	21	15	39
Vegetables[b]	3	2	2	2	2	2	3	8
Fruits[c]	1	1	1	1	1	1	1	1
Meat, salami	48	49	45	45	47	48	50	24
Eggs	1	1	2	2	3	2	2	4
Milk	5	5	5	3	5	6	4	8
Cheese	13	16	16	18	16	13	16	8
Miscellaneous	2	3	4	5	2	7	9	8

[a] 1, Aerobic; 2, Aerobic-anaerobic-alternate; 3, Aerobic-anaerobic-massive; 4, Power; 5, Skill with relevant muscular effort; 6, Skill with little muscular effort.

[b] Including potatoes.

[c] Fresh and canned.

mind of the layman, with a threat to the good function of the liver. This belief is widespread, tenacious, and deeply rooted.

Another instance where general sociocultural factors come into play is the consumption of fish. It is almost absent from the diet of the athlete, and it is consumed in the negligible amount of 26 g/day/person by the average Italian (ISTAT, 1971). Much can be and has been said about the low consumption or total avoidance of fish. This phenomenon has been described in different parts of the world (Simmons, 1974a,b), and deep, far removed ancestral motivations are believed to have a role in producing this attitude; but this field may be more aptly explored by the socioethnologist.

The high consumption of meat, especially red meat from beef, may be associated with the "reinforcing" action commonly attributed to this type of food, both by the athlete and the layman.

In conclusion, the results of this study seem to provide some evidence that the practicing athlete follows a special dietary pattern. The attention of the athlete seems to be concentrated upon relatively few dietary items, the resulting diet being monotonous. Valuable foods may be neglected, ignored, or even intentionally avoided on the extravagant ground that they are deemed to be unsuitable for one or another of the various physical exercises. Finally, the persistence of dietetically improper beliefs and habits, although it does not seem to be conducive to a grossly imbalanced diet, may nevertheless cause unduly high costs of the diet, an unjustifiable waste of extra nutrients, and disappointment when special dietary regimens do not succeed in influencing athletic performance.

When comparing the results of dietary surveys conducted on the Italian athletes who participated in the previous Olympic Games in Rome (1960), Tokyo (1964), and Mexico City (1968), there is evidence of some data showing a lower incidence of dietary mistakes. This fact is related to the advice given to the athletes during their periodical check-up.

REFERENCES

Cho, M., and Fryer, B. A. 1974. What foods do physical education majors and basic nutrition students recommend for athletes? J. Am. Diet. Assoc. 65: 541–544.

Dal Monte, A. 1969. Proposta di una classificazione ad orientamento bimeccanico della attivitá sportive. (A proposal for the biomechanical classification of sports.) Med. Sport 22: 12.

Ferro-Luzzi, A., Caldarone, G., and Topi, G. C. 1976. Dietary habits of Italian athletes. Proc. 1st Int. Symp. "Nutrition and Sport," June 23–25, 1975, Leningrad.

Ferro-Luzzi, A., Topi, G. C., and Caldarone, G. 1975. Consumi alimentari abituali di atleti italiani probabili olimpionici (P.O. 1972). (Habitual dietary intakes of Italian athletes applying for the Olympic Games, 1972.) Med. Sport 28: 109–125.

Gounelle, H., and Berard, L. 1966. Les erreurs alimentaries courantes dans la règion parisienne d'après une enquête menée en milieu sportif. (Current dietary mistakes recorded in a survey carried out among people engaged in sports in the area of Paris.) Bull. I.N.S.E.R.M. 21: 47–56.

INN 1972. Composizione in alcuni principi nutritivi e valore calorico degli alimenti comunemente consumati in Italia. (Energy and nutrient composition of food commonly used in Italy.) Istituto Nazionale della Nutrizione, Roma.

ISTAT 1971. Indagine campionaria sui consumi delle famiglie italiane. Anno 1969. (Sample survey on food consumption of Italian families. Year 1969.) Ist. Centr. Stat. Note e Relazioni, 49.

Mickelsen, O. 1970. Nutrition in athletics. Food Nutr. News 41: 1.

Simmons, F. J. 1974a. Rejection of fish as human food in Africa: A problem in history and ecology. Ecol. Food Nutr. 3: 89–105.

Simmons, F. J. 1974b. Fish as forbidden food: The case of India. Ecol. Food Nutr. 3: 185–201.

S'Jongers, J. J., Dufaux, B., and Anseeuw, J. 1976. Some aspects of the diet of the Belgian athlete. Med. Sport 29: 242–243.

Study of Energy Expenditure and Protein Needs of Top Weight Lifters

K. A. Laritcheva, N. I. Yalovaya, V. I. Shubin, P. V. Smirnov

Many investigations deal with protein metabolism and protein requirements during high and long-term physical loading. Contradictory data in this field make it difficult to ascertain exactly whether the protein needs of the organism change during higher physical activity (Gontzea, Dumitrache, and Schutzescu, 1961; Chailley-Bert et al., 1962; Darden and Schendel, 1971; Mole and Johnson, 1971; Kofranyi, 1972; Shephard, 1973; Cerny, 1975; Consolazio et al., 1975; Durnin, 1975; Eller and Viru, 1975; Shiraki and Joshimura, 1975).

The elaboration of diets ensuring an optimum energy and metabolic balance during physical loads and stress situations in champion sport is impossible without special investigations of energy expenditures and peculiarities of metabolic processes in top athletes, along with investigations in model experiments on animals.

ANIMAL EXPERIMENTS

Experimental data on the influence of both protein deficiency and excess were gained in a laboratory model with male Wistar rats swimming 6 days a week in water 30–32°C (see Table 1 for schedule details). The animals were fed three isocaloric diets with 6, 18, and 30% protein (casein). Control animals were given the same diet without physical loading.

The weight gain was lowest in the animals with the lowest proportion of protein (Table 1); these animals also achieved the lowest (shortest) performance during maximal work loading at the end of the experiment (Table 2). Animals with 18 and 30% protein in their diet differed neither by weight nor maximal performance. Obviously, an increased protein ratio did not improve performance; the nitrogen excretion was increased in the group with 30% protein (328 ± 19.6 mg/24 hr) as compared to the group with 18% protein (190 ± 13.6 mg/24 hr).

Table 1.   Changes in the body weights of rats on diets with different protein contents during the 30-day experimental period

Group	N	Protein content of diet (caloric volume per 100 ml)	Weight gain (g)
1 (Swimming 6 times per week)	9	6	42 ± 3.1^a
2 (Swimming 6 times per week)	31	18	115 ± 4.6
3 (Swimming 6 times per week)	21	30	126 ± 8.6

[a] Differences between groups 2 and 3 are significant ($p < 0.05$). Training scheme: First week—swimming 15–60 min; Second week—swimming 15 min with a load equaling 5% of body weight; Third week—swimming 10 min with a load equaling 7% of body weight.

When comparing experimental animals with the same proportion of protein in their diet (again 6, 18, and 30%) but a different work load (swimming with 7% load either 3 or 6 times a week), an increase of nitrogen excretion was observed in protein deficient rats (i.e., with 6% of protein —see Table 3), which was not true in the other two groups. Creatinine excretion did not depend on the protein content of the diet. The ratio of creatinine nitrogen to total nitrogen in the urine was, therefore, lowest in rats fed the high-protein diet, and highest in protein deficient animals.

Creatine excretion in rats trained 6 times a week did not depend on the protein content of the diet. In less intensively trained rats the excretion of creatine was not observed (Table 3). Lactic and pyruvic acid increased significantly after a work load, but did not differ according to different proportions of protein in the diet.

As follows from this experimental model study, excess protein did not improve maximal performance capacity of swimming rats. In-

Table 2.   Duration of maximum load in rats fed diets with different protein contents

Group of rats	Protein content (caloric volume %)	N	Duration of swimming in min (with a load of 10% body weight)
1	6	9	6.3 ± 1.5^a
2	18	31	18.3 ± 3.5
3	30	21	16.3 ± 4.3

[a] Differences between second and third groups significant ($p < 0.01$), ($p < 0.05$).

Table 3. Effects of physical activity[a] and protein content of diets on 24-hour excretion of total nitrogen, creatine, and creatinine in trained rats.

Group	N	Physical exercise[a] (times per week)	Protein content (caloric volume per 100 ml)	Total nitrogen (mg/24 h)	Creatinine (mg/24 h)	Percent creatinine nitrogen of total nitrogen	Creatine (mg/24 h)
1	9	6	6	150 ± 9.2	5.6 ± 0.5	1.39 ± 0.09	1.11 ± 0.2
2	31	6	18	190 ± 18.6	5.7 ± 0.5	1.10 ± 0.08	1.12 ± 0.2
3	21	6	30	328 ± 29.6	5.0 ± 0.8	0.56 ± 0.01	0.89 ± 0.18
1	8	3	6	70 ± 8.3	4.8 ± 0.6	2.29 ± 0.09	0
2	8	3	18	150 ± 14.8	6.3 ± 0.5	1.56 ± 0.1	0
3	8	3	30	290 ± 35.0	6.1 ± 0.7	0.96 ± 0.05	0

[a] Swimming with a load.

creased excretion of nitrogen because of excess protein can even mean an additional functional loading of the organism.

EXPERIMENT ON WEIGHT LIFTERS

Protein needs were studied directly in champion weight lifters of the USSR. The age of the investigated men ranged from 21 to 34 years, height ranged from 146 to 178 cm, and weight ranged from 54 to 109 kg. The period of weight lifting training spanned 5 to 20 years. All physical loads were expressed relative to 24-hr energy expenditures. The energy values of the main types of the activity, including training, were determined by the method of indirect calorimetry, using an automatic gas analyzer ('Spirolyt—2'). The energy expenditure during sleeping, meals, etc. was calculated from standard tables. The state of protein metabolism was determined from experiments on nitrogen assimilation and balance (Consolazio et al., 1975) and excretion of final products of nitrogen metabolims (urea, creatinine, creatine, amino nitrogen, and ammonia) in urine and sweat (Cerny, 1975).

The authors' investigations showed that in 90–150 min of training and performance of 7,000–17,000 kg, the energy expenditure was equal to 400–1,100 kcal. At higher loads, performance could reach a level of 300,000 kg. In that case energy expenditure may be 1,800 kcal (Table 4). Twenty-four hr energy expenditure in weight lifters ranged between 3,800 and 4,500 kcal, and at high loadings it ranged between 5,000 and 5,200 kcal. The specific energy expenditure during train- and urea content in the blood, sweat, and urine. This was also seen in (about 20%). This expenditure depended on the work performance. A dependence of the efficiency of energy utilization on training intensity

Table 4.   Energy expenditure of athletes during training

Subject	Body weight (kg)	Exercise (kg)	Load (kg)	Training duration (min)	Energy expenditure during training (kcal)
1	52	7,250	7,632	90	470
2	56	6,280	6,810	120	408
3	62	9,570	9,608	165	622
4	74	10,320	10,604	120	549
5	82	16,620	17,320	150	1,080
6	110	27,970	29,820	240	1,818

Table 5.   Nitrogen metabolism of athletes in camps before competitions

Subject	Protein consumption (g/kg of body weight/24 hr)	Nitrogen excretion (g/24 hr)			Nitrogen balance (± g/24 hr)	Assimilation of dietary nitrogen (%)
		Urine	Feces	Total		
1	1.85	18.90	0.87	19.77	−0.88	95.39
2	2.12	28.11	5.86	33.97	+3.13	84.20
3	2.16	21.34	4.95	26.29	+2.10	82.56
4	2.76	23.67	5.95	29.62	+3.06	81.79

and sport level was simultaneously noted. In top athletes, a lower energy output was observed. The period before the start was characterized by a considerable increase in energy output, even in champion athletes. Expenditure during competitions was about 25% higher than during training, with the same performance.

The analysis of the athlete's caloric intake showed that it corresponded to the energy expenditure. However, the nutrient content did not correspond to the principles of balanced diet, possibly because of specific dietary habits of athletes. The values were: protein, 14−18%; fat, 45−48% (which is excessive); and carbohydrates, 41−37%.

Study of the influence of diets with different protein contents on nitrogen assimilation, and the balance and excretion of products of nitrogen metabolism in champion athletes revealed that protein requirements were not identical in various periods of sport activities. Preliminary investigations showed that in the period of preparation for important top-level contests, protein intake corresponded to 2.2−2.6 g/kg of body weight/24 hr. Higher protein levels were not reasonable, because a further increase of protein intake promoted a decrease in its assimilation and retention, and an increase in total nitrogen excretion and urea content in the blood, sweat, and urine. This was also seen in laboratory animals (Table 3). At protein levels of less than 2 g/kg of body weight in some athletes during intensive training, a negative nitrogen balance was observed (Table 5) despite high nitrogen assimilation (95%). During periods when athletes were not exposed to increased physical and psychic stress, a protein intake of 2 g/kg of body weight was enough to sustain the nitrogen balance (Table 6).

In these experiments (Table 5, 6), nitrogen losses by the sweat, skin, hair, and nails were not taken into consideration. During moderate physical activity under normal conditions these losses amount to 0.3−0.5 g/24 hr (Darden and Schendel, 1971; Mole and Johnson, 1971; Kofranyi, 1972). In weight lifters, nitrogen losses in sweat were 3.08 ± 0.65 g/24 hr (Durnin, 1975).

Table 6.   Nitrogen metabolism in athletes between training sessions

Subject	Protein consumption (g/24hr/kg of body weight)	Nitrogen excretion g/24 hr Urine	Feces	Nitrogen balance (± g/24 hr)	Assimilation of dietary nitrogen (%)
1	1.85	13.99	2.21	+1.35	85.1
2	1.36	14.81	2.16	+1.28	88.2
3	1.50	14.0	2.50	+1.74	86.2

The authors' investigations showed that in diets with a 14% protein content, nitrogen excretion by sweat during 1.5 hr training was equal to 1.27 ± 0.18 g, urea excretion was equal to 1.44 ± 0.135g, and ratio of urea nitrogen to total nitrogen in the urine was equal to 56.6 ± 8.5%. To determine protein needs in athletes, it should be taken into consideration that nitrogen assimilation is influenced both by the protein content and energy value of diets. This was ascertained in earlier investigations on healthy young men under strictly controlled conditions. The results indicated that 24-hr energy expenditures corresponded to approximately 2,500–3,000 kcal. It was shown that during a 10-day period a protein content ranging from 1.3 to 1.6 g/kg of body weight/24 hr and a total energy of 2,700 kcal maintained a positive nitrogen balance in all subjects.

It should be noted that when caloric values are identical, a higher protein content in diets corresponds to higher values of positive nitrogen balance (Table 7). The value of nitrogen balance depends on the caloric value of diets. For a diet adequate in energy value (2,700 kcal) and protein content of 2.3 g/kg of body weight, the nitrogen balance is positive. In hypocaloric diets (1,800 kcal) with the same protein content (1.3 g/kg), the nitrogen balance is negative. With low calorie (1,200 kcal) and low protein diets (0.1g/kg), the nitrogen balance is markedly negative (−0.5). Attention should be paid to this dependence of nitrogen balance upon energy value of diets and protein content during periods of excessively reduced diets by weight lifters.

CONCLUSIONS

Despite the large number of investigations devoted to protein requirements of athletes, there is no uniform opinion concerning the optimum dietary level, and this problem still remains unsolved. Coaches and champion athletes in sport disciplines requiring speed and great muscle strength (heavy athletes, throwers, etc.) have traditionally included

Table 7. Nitrogen balance in diets with different caloric and protein content

Subject	Energy value (kcal)	Dietary protein (g)	Dietary protein (g/kg of body weight)	Dietary nitrogen (g)	Urinary nitrogen (g/24 hr)	Nitrogen in feces (g/24 hr)	Nitrogen balance (± g/24 hr)
1	2,700	120.0	1.6	19.2	16.2	1.2	+1.8
2	2,700	100.0	1.3	16.0	14.0	1.3	+0.7
3	1,800	95.0	1.3	15.2	15.8	1.4	−2.0
4	1,200	76.0	1.0	12.2	13.0	1.6	−2.4
5	1,200	6.0	0.1	0.96	5.5	0.46	−5.0

large amounts of protein in daily rations; however, this is not always justified. The protein requirements of athletes are not identical in different periods of their sport activities. During the period of training, which is characterized by high physical activity and the growth of muscle mass, the athlete certainly needs more protein.

As indicated by the preliminary data, during the period of intensive training, a balanced diet corresponds to energy expenditure and the protein requirements of athletes correspond to 2.2–2.6 g/kg body weight. Higher protein levels are useless because assimilation declines with excess protein. Total nitrogen excretion, urea, and amino nitrogen excretion in urine and sweat are raised, and the urea concentration in the blood is also increased.

The consumption of specialized protein preparations by athletes should be controlled by physicians. A dietary protein content of 1.3–2.0 g/kg of body weight is considered sufficient.

REFERENCES

Cerny, F. 1975. Protein metabolism during two hour ergometer exercise. In Metabolic Adaptation to Prolonged Physical Exercise, pp. 232–237. Basel.

Chailley-Bert, P., Plas, F., and Pallard, G. 1962. Le metabolisme protidique an cours de l'effort prolonge. (Protein metabolism during prolonged exercise. Medical press.) Presse Med. 70: (15) 705–707.

Consolazio, C. F., Johnson, H. L., Nelson, R. A., Dramise, J. G., and Skala, J. H. 1975. Protein metabolism during intensive physical training in the young adult. Am. J. Clin. Nutr. 28: 29–35.

Darden, E., and Schendel, H. E. 1971. Dietary protein and muscle building. Schol. Coach 40: 7, 70.

Durnin, V. G. A. 1975. Protein requirements and physical activity. International symposium on sportsmen nutrition, p. 118. Abstracts. Warszava.

Eller, A. K., and Viru, A. A. 1975. Protein metabolism during prolonged exercise. Questions of athletes nutrition. Abstracts of the reports of the International Symposium, pp. 45–46. Leningrad.

Fischer, H. 1967. Nutritional aspects of protein reserves. In A.A. Albanese (ed.), Newer Methods of Nutritional Biochemistry, Vol. 3, pp. 101–181. New York. (1967).

Folin, O. 1905. Laws governing the chemical composition of urine. Am J. Physiol. 13: 66–77.

Gontzea, J., Dumitrache, S., and Schutzescu, P. 1961. Untersuchungen über den mechanismus der vermehrten stickstoffausscheidung durch den harn unter der einwirkung von muskelarbeit. (A study on the mechanism of a rise in nitrogen excretion with urine under the influence of muscle exercise.) Int. Z. Angew. Physiol. Einschl. Arbeitsphysiol. 19: 7–17.

Kofranyi, E. 1972. Protein and amino acid requirement. A. Nitrogen balance in adults. In E. J. Bigwood (ed.), Protein and Amino Acid Function, pp. 1–61. Pergamon Press, Oxford.

Kremer, Ju. M. 1965. Biochemistry of Protein Nutrition, pp. 172–182. Sinante. Riga.

Mole, P. A., and Johnson, R. E. 1971. Disclosure by dietary modification of an exercise—induced protein catabolism in man. J. Appl. Physiol. 31: 185–190.

Munro, H. N. 1972. Amino acid requirements and utilization by individual mammalian tissues. In E.J. Bigwood (ed.), Protein and Amino Acid Functions, pp. 157–196. Pergamon Press, Oxford.

Patwardhan, V. N. 1961. Utilization of vegetable and animal protein in human subjects. In Proteins and Amino Acid in Nutrition, 5th International Congress of Nutrition. Panel 11, Washington, pp. 20, 73–80.

Pokrovsky, A. A. (Ed.). 1969. Biochemical methods of investigations in clinic (Guide). Medicine, Moscow.

Shephard, P. J. 1973. Physical activity and metabolism. Role of exercise biochemistry in sports medicine. J. Sports Med. Phys. Fitness 13: 45–53.

Shiraki, K., and Joshimura. 1975. Anemia during strenuous muscular exercise (sport anemia). J. Postgrad. Med. 21 (suppl. 30).

Vysotsky, V. G., Sokolov, V. N., and Jatzyshina, T. A. 1976. Concepzija labilnogo belca i adaptazija azotistogo obmena pri belcovoi nedostatotschnosti u tscheloveca. (The concept of labile protein and adaptation of nitrogen metabolism with protein deficiency in man.) J. Voprosy Pitaniya N4: 29–36.

Nutrition and Occupational Activities in Developed and Developing Countries

Nutrition, Physical Activity, and Physical Fitness in Contrasting Environments

N. G. Norgan, A. Ferro-Luzzi

In the industrialized countries, there is concern about present-day levels of physical activity and physical fitness. It is believed that there has been a recent trend to a sedentary way of life, resulting in low levels of activity and fitness, which contrasts sharply with the active lives of earlier generations to which man may have become genotypically adapted. Just as there are optimal levels of nutrition for health, there may be optimal levels of physical activity for physical fitness and health. The evidence is not unequivocal. Edholm (1970) has questioned the assumption that levels of physical activity have decreased in the United Kingdom over the last 100 years, and Keys (1970), in critically appraising the evidence for a relationship between levels of physical activity and coronary heart disease, has pleaded for more rigourously designed studies to clarify the issue.

In developing countries, high levels of manual work are regarded as common, and although planes of nutrition are low, they are often adequate. Nevertheless, physical fitness is not particularly high. There are some populations renowned for their physical fitness and endurance, but it is not clear whether these arise through environmental (nutrition, physical activity) or genetic factors.

The relative importance of these factors and the validity of the widely held belief of a relationship between habitual physical activity and physical fitness may be examined by comparing different occupational and cultural groups.

DEFINITIONS AND INDICES

Level of Nutrition

It is important to focus attention on energy intakes in the present context because it is recognized that the protein contents of all diets and most staple foodstuffs are adequate if energy requirements are met (Payne, 1975). Individually weighed food intakes are regarded as most accurate (± 10%), although in many areas food composition data are scarce.

Habitual Physical Activity

Daily energy expenditure is the common objective measure of habitual physical activity. Diary records of activity with measured energy cost of activities may have an accuracy of ± 15%. Similar daily energy expenditures can occur with entirely different patterns of habitual physical activity. Peak activity is important for a training effect.

Physical Fitness

Physical fitness can be regarded as the response to exercise or the capacity for exercise. The most common single criterion is the maximum oxygen uptake ($\dot{V}O_2$ max). It reflects the overall capacity of the cardiorespiratory system and the musculature to transport and utilize oxygen and to expend energy. Groups of different body sizes are compared by expressing $\dot{V}O_2$ max as ml O_2/kg body weight/min. Because many "primitive" groups have low fat contents and therefore proportionately more lean tissue, results may need to be standardized more thoroughly. Habituation and mode of exercise effect the determined value (Shephard et al., 1968a). In many population groups, $\dot{V}O_2$ max is difficult to measure directly, but is predicted from submaximal data (Shephard et al., 1968b) with a decrease in accuracy (Davies, 1968). $\dot{V}O_2$ max has an important genetic component, and Cotes and Davies (1969) have argued that level of fitness should be regarded as the proportion of endowment utilized.

NUTRITION, ACTIVITY, AND FITNESS IN ITALIAN SHIPYARD WORKERS

The interrelations between nutrition, activity, and fitness in developed countries are illustrated by a study conducted on a sample of the 6,000 shipyard workers of ItalCantieri, Monfalcone, Italy. In shipyards there are a variety of occupations, ranging from clerical and administrative jobs to heavy physical activity, often combined with skilled tasks. A nonrandom sample was selected to include a wide variety of occupations that were grouped into three grades of severity: light, medium, and heavy. This classification was made after meetings with the workers and after observation and inspection of the workers and work sites, but before measurements of energy cost of activities and occupations were made. The light work category included clerks, crane drivers, and workshop mechanics. The main difference between the medium and heavy categories was the place of work; working on board in cramped conditions and having to manhandle heavy equipment and scale ladders frequently were considered examples of the heaviest work.

The subjects were of Italian origin and lived locally. They underwent a medical examination before the study began. The three activity groups did not differ in physical characteristics (Table 1).

Dietary intakes and daily energy expenditure were determined over 7 consecutive days in 150 subjects. Dietary intakes were determined by the individual inventory method using Italian tables of food composition (Fidanza, 1974). Daily energy expenditure was calculated from 24-hr diary records of activity, and the energy cost of tasks was determined by indirect calorimetry (Durnin and Brockway, 1959). Measurements of body composition and response to exercise were made in 132 of the subjects.

Body density was measured by underwater weighing (Durnin and Rahaman, 1967) with the simultaneous determination of lung residual volume (Rahn, Fenn, and Otis, 1949). Percentage of body weight as fat was calculated by substitution in Siri's equation (Siri, 1956). Submaximal exercise tests, using a double 23 cm step or bicycle ergometer, were continuous with four work loads to elicit heart rates of $110-160$ beats/min, depending on age. The subjects exercised at each work load for 3 min, and recordings of cardiac frequency (fC) and oxygen consumption ($\dot{V}_{O_2}$) were made over the 3rd min using standard methods (Weiner and Lourie, 1969). These values were plotted and a line of best fit drawn through them. Cardiac frequencies at given oxygen uptakes, e.g., fC 1.0, and oxygen uptakes at given cardiac frequencies, e.g., $\dot{V}_{O_2}$ 150, were read off. The predicted maximum oxygen uptake, $\dot{V}_{O_2}$ max,

Table 1.   The physical characteristics of Italian shipyard workers

Category of work	N		Age (years)	Height (cm)	Weight (kg)	Fat-free mass (kg)
Light	38	$\bar{X}$	35.7	174.3	75.6	58.3
		SD	8.5	5.2	9.7	6.0
Medium	37	$\bar{X}$	39.3	172.3	77.9	59.7
		SD	9.7	5.1	11.3	7.3
Heavy	75	$\bar{X}$	37.3	172.9	76.1	58.7
		SD	7.9	7.2	13.4	7.5

was taken at the fC max for the age group of each subject (Andersen et al., 1971). Values for fC 1.0 and 1.5 and predicted $\dot{V}_{O_2}$ max in 22–29-year-olds obtained by this extrapolation procedure were not significantly different from those obtained using nomograms (Åstrand and Rodahl, 1970; Cotes et al., 1973a).

Dietary Intakes

The intakes of nutrients and energy are shown in Table 2. Protein intakes, two-thirds of which were of animal origin, averaged 100 g/day, 1.3 g/kg body weight. Fat intakes were 128 g/day, with a slight preponderance of animal fats. The alcohol intakes of 54 g/day represented 12% of the total energy intake, and fat and protein contributed 36% and 12%, respectively. The mean daily energy intake was 3,211 kcal (42 kcal/kg), but energy intakes differed between the three work categories: light, 3,028± 549 (mean ±SD) (40 kcal/kg); medium, 3,181 ± 466 (41 kcal/kg); heavy, 3,324 ± 649 (44 kcal/kg). Nutrient intakes differed in the same way as energy intakes. These dietary intakes are indicative of an adequately nourished sample pursuing moderately active work.

Dietary intakes did not vary much with age over the range 22–49 years. Subjects aged 40 to 49 years were 5 kg heavier than the younger individuals, so intakes per kg body weight were lower. Alcohol intakes were higher in this group: 65 g/day, 14% of energy intake. The 11 subjects age 50 to 56 years had the lowest energy intakes 2849 ± 417 (39 kcal/kg).

Energy Expenditures

Mean daily energy expenditure agreed well with the mean daily energy intakes, with a difference of 62 kcal/day (Table 3). However, the energy expenditures do suggest greater differences in activity between the groups than energy intakes, and support the method of activity classification. The light activity energy expenditure of 38 kcal/kg identifies the group as sedentary workers, and the heavy activity group, 43 kcal/kg, would be regarded as moderately active (FAO/WHO, 1973). The differences in energy expenditure arise from the different demand of occupations. Nonoccupational energy expenditure was constant, 1,570 kcal, but energy expenditure in working hours was 1,295, 1,641, and 1,915 kcal in light, medium, and heavy groups—a 25% and 50% greater expenditure in the medium and heavy groups. Thus the three groups show clear differences in physical activity, particularly at work.

The relation of energy expenditure to age was similar to that of energy intake. There was no difference (3,160–3,180 kcal/day) in the

Table 2. Mean daily energy and nutrient intakes of Italian shipyard workers

Category of work	N		Body weight (kg)	Energy/day (kcal)	(kcal/kg)	Protein/day (g)	(g/kg)	Fat/day (g)	Carbohydrate/day (g)	Alcohol/day (g)
Light	38	X̄	75.6	3,028	40	93.7	1.24	121.9	329.6	45.1
		SD	9.7	549		18.5		29.8	79.3	26.4
Medium	37	X̄	77.9	3,181	41	102.4	1.31	123.6	336.8	55.7
		SD	11.3	466		12.5		24.2	82.0	34.0
Heavy	75	X̄	76.1	3,324	44	105.2	1.38	132.9	346.8	56.8
		SD	13.4	649		21.9		30.0	79.1	34.1

Table 3. Mean daily energy expenditures of Italian shipyard workers

Type of activity	N	Body weight (kg)	Energy intake (kcal)	Energy expenditure (kcal)	(kcal/kg)	Difference (kcal)	Energy expenditure on working days (kcal)	(kcal/kg)	Energy expenditure during working hours (kcal)
Light	38	75.6	3,028	2,855	38	+173	2,857	38	1,295
Medium	36	77.9	3,181	3,137	40	+44	3,245	42	1,641
Heavy	75	76.1	3,324	3,309	43	+15	3,488	46	1,915
Mean	149	76.4	3,214	3,152	41	+62	3,268	43	1,691

three age groups 22–49 years. Older subjects had lower expenditures, 2,885 kcal/day.

As it is to be expected, a number of activities involved considerable expenditures of energy. Over 1,000 measurements of the energy cost of 65 different active work and leisure tasks were made, 12 tasks of which involved energy expenditures greater than 5 kcal/min/65 kg man.

Responses to Exercise

Influence of Age   The response to submaximal exercise in these subjects did not seem to be influenced by age. The $\dot{V}O_2$ at fC 150 was similar in the four age groups (Table 4). The older age group had slightly higher $\dot{V}O_2$ 150 ml/kg/min, but there were a small number of subjects. Similarly, cardiac frequencies at standard $\dot{V}O_2$ did not vary much. This suggests that fitness was independent of age. Allowing for fat-free mass by using a linear regression equation calculated for these subjects, fC 1.5 of 22–39-year-olds was similar to that of United Kingdom factory workers (Cotes, 1976).

A possible explanation for the apparent maintenance of fitness with age in these industrial workers could be that the nature of the work has changed. Although older workers may have experienced several years of heavy physical activity and, indeed, may have selected themselves for such occupations, younger workers have the benefits of automation and the application of ergonomics, and this exhibits itself in lower levels of fitness in the younger working population. Many of the older workers recalled the greater effort required to rivet plates by hammering compared to modern welding techniques. An alternative explanation is a fall in cardiac frequency at a constant oxygen uptake with age. This has been demonstrated satisfactorily in women (Cotes et al., 1973b). However, the composition of the age groups was not standardized for work category or body composition.

Predicted $\dot{V}O_2$ max declined with age, as is to be expected with the extrapolation procedure. In the 22–29 year age group, $\dot{V}O_2$ ml/kg/min was low (38.5 ml/kg/min), and it compared unfavorably with other groups (Cumming, 1967; Shephard, 1967; Cotes et al., 1969). Prediction procedures usually underestimate $\dot{V}O_2$ max in untrained subjects (Åstrand and Rodahl, 1970), and this may explain the similar submaximal exercise responses but different $\dot{V}O_2$ max in these subjects compared to United Kingdom factory workers. Davies (1968) has proposed correcting predicted values to give a more realistic estimate. Using his equation, $\dot{V}O_2$ max of 22–29-year-olds is increased by 0.43 liters to 3.35 liters. Cotes et al. (1969) found predicted $\dot{V}O_2$ max of the factory workers to be underestimated by 0.3 liters. Therefore, the results of the two groups are essentially similar.

Table 4. Analysis of oxygen consumption ($\dot{V}O_2$) and cardiac frequencies (fC) from submaximal exercise tests

Age group (years)	N	Body weight (kg)	Fat-free mass (kg)	$\dot{V}O_2$ at fC 150 (liters/min)	$\dot{V}O_2$ at fC max (liters/min)	$\dot{V}O_2$ at fC max (ml/kg/min)	fC at $\dot{V}O_2$ 1.5 (beats/min)
22–29	30	76.1 9.0	61.6 5.9	1.99	2.92	38.5	127.5
30–39	57	74.9 12.9	58.4[a] 7.5	1.97	2.77	37.5	128.5
40–49	38	78.5 11.6	57.6[a] 6.6	2.03	2.60[a]	33.6[b]	124.3
50–56	7	69.5 11.0	52.6[c] 5.5	1.99	2.41[b]	35.4	125.5

[a] Significance of the difference from 22–29-year-olds: $p < 0.05$.
[b] $p < 0.01$.
[c] $p < 0.001$.

Category of Work   The responses to exercise of the three work categories are shown in Table 5. The mean ages differed only slightly. The medium work activity group members were 2−2.5 kg heavier, with slightly greater fat-free mass (FFM) and fat mass. Cardiac frequency at $\dot{V}O_2$ 1.0 and 1.5 were lower, and $\dot{V}O_2$ at fC 150 were higher in this group. Predicted $\dot{V}O_2$ max was similar to the heavy work group, as ml/kg weight/min or ml/kg FFM/min. These two groups had higher maximal values than the light activity group, although only the medium work group exhibited a significant difference ($p < 0.05$).

Body Weight and Body Composition   Body weight showed an insignificant increase with age, but FFM and fat mass altered progressively with age, −1.9 kg and +2.9 kg per decade ($p < 0.01$). Fat-free mass showed the highest correlation with exercise parameters ($r = 0.50−0.60$) and, by multiple regression step analysis, the degree of correlation was not markedly improved by adding in age, height, weight, fat mass, or any combination of these.

When subjects are grouped according to body density (Table 5), differences in body weight and weight of fat are evident. Body weight in the obese group (density < 1.0365, %fat > 27.5) was on the average 85.9 kg, 130% of desirable weight for height compared with 69.2 kg in the normal group. However, mean FFM of the three groups was similar, as were submaximal exercise parameters. Oxygen consumptions at fC 150/kg FFM were 33.7, 34.3, and 34.1 ml/kg FFM/min in the normal, plump, and obese groups. $\dot{V}O_2$ max were also similar. In this instance, expressing results as ml/kg weight/min clearly penalizes heavy subjects, and suggests an unfavorable cardiorespiratory response with increasing adiposity.

In conclusion, the responses to submaximal exercise and predicted $\dot{V}O_2$ max in these groups of contrasting physical activity were similar except for the light and medium work groups.

NUTRITION, ACTIVITY, AND FITNESS IN NEW GUINEANS

Papua-New Guinea was uninfluenced by Western contacts until recent times. The way of life is changing and will continue to change. At present, most of the adults are subsistence horticulturalists. From 1969−1971 a study of the nutritional status, energy expenditure, and body composition of two contrasting communities was conducted (Norgan, Ferro-Luzzi, and Durnin, 1974). This was part of an International Biological Programme (IBP) multidisciplinary study on human adaptability in a tropical ecosystem (Harrison and Walsh, 1974). The first community was the Kaul villages on a small fertile island off the north coast, fairly typical of coastal populations. The second group,

Table 5. Exercise responses according to category of work and body composition

	Work category			Body composition		
				Density: >	Normal 1.0530	Plump 1.0530–1.0365	Obese <1.0365
				Percent fat: <	20	20–27.5	>27.5
Characteristics	Light	Medium	Heavy		Normal	Plump	Obese
	($N = 35$)	($N = 34$)	($N = 63$)		($N = 50$)	($N = 58$)	($N = 24$)
Age (years)	35.6	38.0	36.6		33.1	37.8	41.4
Weight (kg)	74.9	77.6	75.5		69.2	77.5	85.9
Height (cm)	174.1	173.0	173.1		172.7	174.3	172.3
Density (g/ml)	1.0491	1.0468	1.0490		1.0617	1.0452	1.0288
Fat-free mass (kg)	58.1	59.4	58.5		57.8	59.2	59.0
$\dot{V}O_2$ at fC 150 (liters/min)	1.87[b]	2.16	1.98[a]		1.95	2.03	2.01
$\dot{V}O_2$ at fC max (liters/min)	2.58[a]	2.89	2.76		2.75	2.77	2.69
$\dot{V}O_2$ at fC max (ml/kg/min)	34.7[a]	37.7	37.2		39.8	36.1[b]	31.3[c]
fC at $\dot{V}O_2$ 1.5 (beats/min)	132.4[a]	118.8	127.6[a]		129.3	124.5	126.1

[a] Significance of the differences in exercise responses from medium work category or from normal body composition group: $p < 0.05$.
[b] $p < 0.01$.
[c] $p < 0.001$.

Lufa, was a highland (1,800 m) community, typical of much of New Guinea. Both groups were subsistence horticulturalists, but some cash crops were grown and a few adult males were in paid employment. The Lufans had had less contact with Europeans. The way of life and general environment of the two groups has been described by Norgan, Ferro-Luzzi, and Durnin (1974).

The subjects were small in stature (160 cm), of low body weight (57 kg), and of low fat content (10%), compared to European populations. Obesity was absent and good muscular development was the norm in adults. All groups showed significant decreases in body weight with age, except Kaul males. This is the reverse of the situation pertaining in developed countries. Dietary intakes and energy expenditures were measured using the techniques described for the ItalCantieri study.

Nutrition

Vegetables were the staple foodstuffs in both groups. In Kaul, taro (*Colocasia* and *Xanthosoma*) supplied 42% of the energy and 24% of the protein intakes. Total protein intakes were 0.66 and 0.53 g/kg in men and women, 98% and 77% of safe levels of intake (FAO/WHO, 1973). Energy was derived predominantly from carbohydrate: protein calories were 6.5% and fat calories 17.5% of the energy intakes. Energy intakes were low, considering the way of life, 35 kcal/kg for men and 31 kcal/kg for women, and do not reach recommended intakes for light workers (FAO/WHO, 1973). Store foods contributed 21% of the energy intakes and 29% of protein intakes.

In Lufa, the staple sweet potato *(Ipomea batatas)* assumed more importance, contributing 64% of the energy intake and 37% of the protein intake. Total protein intakes were higher (0.85 g/kg) and more adequate (120% and 150% of safe levels for men and women), and provided 6.5−7.2% of the energy. Energy intakes were 44 and 41 kcal/kg, approaching the recommended levels for moderately active workers. Store foods contributed significantly less to energy and protein intakes, 10% and 15% respectively, but in amounts greater than described previously, demonstrating the changing way of life.

Hence, the diets were adequate but the plane of nutrition would be considered low, particularly for protein and fat.

Energy Expenditure

A careful study was made of the activity of most of the dietary subjects over five consecutive days. A total of 1,160 measurements of energy expenditure were made on the various activities of the subjects, and total daily energy expenditures were calculated. They are given in Table 6 with the dietary intakes of the *same* subjects. Highland men and young Kaul men had energy expenditures that were similar (45

Table 6. Mean daily intakes and expenditure of energy of New Guineans

Society and age (years)	N	Body weight (kg)	Energy intake			Energy expenditure		
			(kcal/day)	(kcal/kg/day)	(kcal/day)	(kcal/kg/day)	(kcal/65 kg)[a]
Kaul men							
18–29	17	57.7	2,153	37.3	2,619	45.4	2,950
30–48	25	55.3	1,907	34.5	2,162	39.1	2,541
Lufa men							
18–29	25	58.8	2,482	42.2	2,567	43.7	2,838
30–49	15	56.0	2,609	46.6	2,577	46.0	2,991
							(kcal/55 kg)[b]
Kaul women							
18–29	23	49.8	1,411	28.3	1,932	38.8	2,133
30–49	17	45.9	1,459	31.8	1,692	36.9	2,027
Lufa women							
18–29	31	51.1	2,099	41.1	2,268	44.4	2,441
30–49	7	46.3	2,150	46.4	2,141	46.2	2,543

[a] For men.
[b] For women.

kcal/kg) and indicative of moderate physical activity (FAO/WHO, 1973). Older Kaul men had levels similar to light workers (39 kcal/kg). There was a large difference in the energy expenditure of the women (Lufa, 45 kcal/kg; Kaul, 38 kcal/kg), and Lufa women were moderately to very active. When adjusted to standard body weights, the energy expenditures are similar to those of many European occupations (Durnin and Passmore, 1967). Energy intakes and expenditures of the Kauls differ; possible explanations have been considered (Norgan, Ferro-Luzzi, and Durnin, 1974). Hipsley and Kirk (1965) found even lower values in a small number of coastal and highland men (35–38 kcal/kg/day), but values in women were similar to those above.

Energy expenditure decreased with age in Kauls, but not in Lufans. Expressed as kcal/kg/day to allow for the decreases in body weight with age, the decrease was significant ($p < 0.001$) in Kaul males. Expenditures actually increased with age in Lufans, although not significantly.

The diary records confirm that the way of life as unexacting. Most of the day (70%) was spent lying, sitting, or standing. Walking occupied 10% of the 24 hr and was the most important single active task in contributing to the total energy expenditure (20% in Kaul, 27% in Lufa). In Kaul, some of the walking time was spent sauntering around the village, but in the highlands walking often involved climbing steep slopes. Food producing activities, excluding walking to the gardens but including hunting and cash cropping, occupied 3.0–3.5% of the day in Kaul, and 6.0–7.5% in Lufa.

The energy cost of individual tasks shows that some tasks involved moderate energy expenditure (Norgan, Ferro-Luzzi, and Durnin, 1974), but the way of life required only moderate physical activity.

Responses to Exercise

In view of the simple way of life of these people and the relative ease of attaining their basic material needs, their levels of fitness are of considerable interest. The responses to submaximal exercise on a bicycle ergometer in a representative sample of young adults, some of whom also participated in the dietary and activity investigations, has been determined using reliable techniques (Cotes, Anderson, and Patrick, 1974). Cardiac frequencies at oxygen consumptions of 1.0 and 1.5 liters/min were standardized to FFM of 55 kg for men and 40 kg for women by the authors. Cardiac frequencies (fC 1.5 st/min) were 119 in Kauls and 113 in highlanders, compared to 132 in United Kingdom factory workers doing fairly heavy work and 131 in Italian shipyard workers. These responses suggest predicted $\dot{V}_{O_2}$ max of over 55ml/kg/min in Kauls and about 65 ml/kg/min in highlanders. For women, fC

1.0 st/min were 135 in Kaul and 122 in highlands, compared with 134 in United Kingdom factory workers.

New Guinea highlanders have significantly superior responses to coastal men and women, a result that was not ascribed to differences in altitude, and both have lower cardiac frequencies than European factory workers. Cotes (1976) considers differences in physical activity rather than ethnic differences to be important, while recognizing that there are no marked differences in activity of the New Guinean men.

Summary

These two studies do not support the belief that habitual physical activity and fitness are positively related. Higher levels of physical activity in the European shipyard workers were not associated with higher levels of fitness, with one exception. Differences in physical fitness in New Guineans were not associated with differences in level of physical activity. This was also true for the shipyard workers in medium and heavy occupations compared to the New Guineans, where the differences in fitness were more striking.

It is of interest to reappraise some of the evidence that suggests that the level of habitual physical activity is an important determinant of physical fitness.

LEVELS OF HABITUAL
PHYSICAL ACTIVITY RELATED TO FITNESS

Simple Technological Societies

Physical Activity   Few primitive societies unaffected by western technology exist today, but some groups provide evidence that hunter-gatherers are able to meet their material needs without much physical effort (Sahlins, 1974), even though the areas they now occupy represent less favorable habitats. Australian aborigines spend 17 hr/day sitting or lying (McCarthy and McArthur, 1960), and Kalahari Bushmen hunt or gather food for 2−3 days per week (Lee, 1968). Dietary intake data suggest that the energy expenditure of the latter is 2,200−2,400 kcal/day, 50 kcal/kg. Dobe bushmen (Southwest Africa) and the Hazda (Tanzania) spend 2−3 hr/day in food quest activities (Woodburn, 1968; Scudder, 1971).

Shifting cultivators represent a more advanced type of food acquisition: gardens are cleared in forest or bush and then abandoned after one or two seasons. Sufficient food can be produced without excessive effort: 1.5−3.5 hr/day in Philippine swidden rice cultivators (Conklin, 1957), and 1−2 hr/day in New Guineans (Hipsley and Kirk,

1965; Rappaport, 1967; Lea, 1970), involving energy expenditures of 2,500 kcal/day and 45 kcal/kg/day.

Peasant farmers are the next step up in the complexity of food producing activities. They represent the majority of the world population and therefore show a range of ways of life. Gorou (1966) and Clark and Haswell (1970) have summarized much of the available data, and have found that the average time spent in active tasks is 2.5–4.5 hr/day. This is affected by season in most instances, e.g., in the Camerouns the average was as high as 10 hr/day, over a 3-month period.

Within any area higher levels of activity may be found, but these are more common in groups with paid employment: for example, Indian stone cutters and cotton mill workers, energy expenditure 3,050 kcal/day, 65 kcal/kg (Durnin and Passmore, 1967); Nepalese porters, energy intake 3,500 kcal/day (Pugh, 1966); Central American farm employees, energy expenditure 3,690 kcal/day, 61 kcal/kg (Viteri et al., 1971); Columbian sugar cane cutters, 3,426 kcal/day, 58 kcal/kg (Spurr, Barac-Nieto, and Maksud, 1975).

Unfortunately, but not unexpectedly, there is not much reliable and precise information on daily energy expenditure in developing communities or countries. The number of studies combining measurements of dietary intake, energy expenditure, and capacity for exercise are even fewer. However, Shephard and colleagues have performed such comprehensive investigations on Eskimos in the eastern Canadian Arctic. Before examining these, the available data on fitness in developing countries are examined.

Aerobic Power   The information on aerobic power in different ethnic groups has been reviewed (Cumming, 1967; Davies et al., 1972). Representative values of groups following various ways of life are shown in Table 7.

The aerobic power of untrained Caucasian adults shows some variation, but 40–45 ml/kg/min can be taken as the range of values commonly found. Studies by several authors fall in this range (Davies et al., 1972), and this agrees with most of the data quoted by Cumming (1967) and the findings of Andersen (1966) on Norwegians.

Clearly, most of the values found in developing countries are not exceptional, and differences between groups are less than intersubject differences within groups. Yoruba factory workers (56 ml/kg/min) and Canadian Eskimos (59 ml/kg/min) seem to be distinct. Tarahumaras Indian runners have exceptionally high values (63 ml/kg/min) and are reported as having very high energy expenditures (Aghemo, Limas, and Sassi, 1971). They may represent an athletic group that has taken up this activity because of superior endowment, although there is no direct evidence for this.

Table 7. Aerobic power in various cultural groups

Cultural group	N	$\dot{V}_{O_2}$ max ml/kg/min	Literature source
Hunters-gatherers and nomads			
Eskimos	8	44	Andersen, 1966
Arctic Indians	8	49	Andersen, 1966
Nomadic Lapps	16	54	Andersen, 1966
Canadian Eskimos	27	59	Rode and Shephard, 1971
Bushmen	10	47	Wyndham, 1967
Dorobo and Turkana		46	di Prampero and Cerretelli, 1969
Farmers, peasants, and agricultural workers			
Bantu mine recruits	20	45	Wyndham et al., 1966
American Negro sharecroppers		50	Cumming, 1967
Easter Islanders		42	Andersen, 1967a
Tarahumaras Indians	30	39	Aghemo, Limas, and Sassi, 1971
Jamaican hill farmers	19	47	Miller et al., 1972
Yoruba	7	49	Davies et al., 1972
Kurds	19	44	Davies et al., 1972
Yemenites	20	47	Davies et al., 1972
East African sugar cane cutters	19	48	Davies, 1973
Columbian sugar cane cutters	55	45	Maksud, Spurr, and Barac-Nieto, 1976
Urban and nonagricultural workers			
Bantu miners	20	46	Wyndham et al., 1966
Yoruba factory workers	13	56	Davies et al., 1972
Trinidadian clerks and storekeepers	24	37	Miller et al., 1972
Tanzanian, urban	26	47	Davies et al., 1973

Activity times given above suggest that levels of energy expenditure and habitual physical activity may not be particularly high, but this would not be the case for all these groups. Thus the energy expenditure of Jamaican hill farmers is reported as 3,250 kcal/day, 53 kcal/kg/day (Miller et al., 1972). However, in this group and in Columbian sugar cane cutters (energy expenditure 58 kcal/kg/day), aerobic powers are not high.

Response to Submaximal Exercise   The responses to submaximal exercise of different ethnic groups have been compared (Cotes et al., 1974; Cotes, 1976). Cardiac frequencies at $\dot{V}_{O_2}$ 1.5 liters/min, standardized for body composition (FFM) and ambient temperature, increased in this order: New Guinea highlanders (109), Nepalese Gurkhas (113), United Kingdom amateur racing cyclists (114), New Guinea coastal villagers (117), Jamaican farmers (120), Rajputs (122), South Indian servicemen (127), Trinidadian clerks and storekeepers (128), United Kingdom factory workers (132), and Indian civilians (141).

Mean daily energy expenditures were: New Guinea highlanders, 2,567 kcal/day, 44 kcal/kg; New Guinea coastal villagers, 2,619 kcal, 45 kcal/kg; and Jamaicans, 3,250 kcal, 53 kcal/kg. In these subjects the correspondence between the response to submaximal exercise and habitual physical activity is not evident. In addition, differences in $\dot{V}_{O_2}$ max were found between Trinidadians and United Kingdom factory workers with similar cardiac frequencies (Edwards et al., 1972).

It is difficult to agree at this stage with Cotes (1976), that differences in standardized cardiac frequencies are associated with or reflect differences in levels of physical activity, but not ethnic origin.

Eskimos

Activity   Godin and Shephard (1973) have described the activity patterns of the Eskimos in the eastern Canadian Arctic. Although their way of life is changing, about one-third of the food needs in the community of Igloolik were met by the hunt. Twenty-nine of the 113 men were active hunters who used dog teams and mechanized transport. Hunting involved high daily energy expenditures: 2,500–4,400 kcal/day, depending on the type of hunting. The simple average is 3,670 kcal/day, but Rode and Shephard (1971) quote 3,200 kcal as the daily caloric cost of a hunting expedition. Hunting trips may last several weeks in winter, but Godin and Shephard consider that three days per week may be representative overall. If energy expenditure on hunting days were 3,200–3,670 kcal and 2,500–2,700 kcal on non-hunting days, the daily energy expenditure would be 2,800–3,100 kcal per day (42–47 kcal/kg).

A similar number of subjects pursued paid employment around the settlement, and average daily energy expenditure was quoted as 3,300 kcal/day. This was calculated by dividing the day into periods of work, sleep, leisure, etc. and taking an average energy cost. The average energy expenditure for 8 hr of work was taken to be 3.4 kcal/min, the mean of 25 activities measured. Settlement workers may not be employed permanently, and the authors considered four working days per week as typical. Average daily energy expenditure over the year would then be 2,960–3,040 kcal/day (42–43 kcal/kg). These figures are in agreement with those for the overall energy expenditure of the community (Shephard, 1974). In 14 Eskimo women observed for part of the day, calculated energy expenditure was 2,500 kcal/day.

From dietary intake data, Schaefer, quoted by Godin and Shephard (1973), has estimated mean energy expenditures of 2,860, 2,540, and 2,790 kcal in more primitive settlements, and 2,100 kcal/day in the urban community of Frobisher Bay. These values may be taken to represent the average energy expenditure of hunting and non-hunting days.

These figures are not indicative of regular high levels of habitual physical activity; they would fall within the moderately active category (FAO/WHO, 1973). Rode and Shephard (1971) noted that "the immediate impression of Eskimo life is one of leisure and long periods of waiting: activity is brief and intense."

Aerobic Power   Shephard and Rode (1973) and Shephard (1974) have reviewed the available data on the fitness of Arctic communities, and have considered the possible effects of methodological differences, motivation, tuberculosis, and episodic malnutrition. Their results on Igloolik Eskimos are 10−15% higher than previous estimates of other communities, and are regarded as indicative of better techniques, community health, and nutrition. Measured $\dot{V}o_2$ max was 3.5 liters/min in subjects making a good effort (52 ml/kg/min) (Shephard, 1974), compared with a predicted $\dot{V}o_2$ max of 3.7 liters/min. In 20−29-year-old subjects without tb, predicted values were 4.1 liters/min (60 ml/kg/min) (Rode and Shephard, 1971). It is not clear which values should be taken as representative (Shephard, 1976, quotes 52 ml/kg/min), but the authors feel Igloolik Eskimos remain superior to other Eskimo groups and typical Europeans.

Differences in predicted aerobic power between hunters and urbanized individuals were observed: 3.7 liters/min (57 ml/kg/min) and 3.4 liters/min (51 ml/kg/min), respectively. Hunters making 10 or more major expeditions per year had higher aerobic capacities than those who made three or four trips: 62 versus 55 ml/kg/min (Shephard, 1974). Shephard and Rode (1973) noted that these differences cannot be reconciled with the similarity in energy expenditures, but they regarded the substantially higher values in Eskimos compared with "white" communities to reflect, in part, differences in physical activity. They also reported similar predicted $\dot{V}o_2$ max in summer and winter in both activity types. It might be expected that activity would be reduced in winter because of shorter days and inclement weather, but these factors could just as well increase the cost of activity. However, Sinclair (1953) described winter seal hunting of Igloolik Eskimos as characteristic of the so-called "maupoq" (waiting) hunting, where "the hunter sits absolutely still on a block of snow in the raw cold of a short winter day."

Again, the relationship between habitual physical activity and fitness is unclear both within these people and when they are compared to Caucasians with similar activity levels.

Western Societies

Habitual Physical Activity and Aerobic Power   The literature relating habitual physical activity and aerobic power is confused. This seems to result from problems in the assessment of habitual physical activity. Activity patterns and daily energy expenditures have been reviewed (Durnin, 1967; Durnin and Passmore, 1967). There is considerable variation, with occupation often the most influential factor (FAO/WHO, 1973; Durnin, 1975). Within any group, the levels of nonoccupational activity may vary and reduce the magnitude of the differences between occupations. This reduces the usefulness of job description as an indicator of habitual physical activity and has led to a certain amount of circular reasoning in relating physical activity levels to fitness. When differences in $\dot{V}O_2$ max exist, then differences in activity are often assumed or supported by subjective classification, but when $\dot{V}O_2$ max are similar, these are assumed to result, in part, from similar levels of activity.

Thus, Davies et al. (1972), in considering ethnic differences in physical work capacity, divided groups into primitive, inactive, and active categories within which $\dot{V}O_2$ max ml/kg/min tend to be similar: primitive, 46–50; inactive, 40–47; and active, 52–56. One wonders if descriptions of activity were made on the basis of $\dot{V}O_2$ max rather than activity, as the authors note: "In the main, the Kurds and Yemenites were active agricultural workers, whereas the Caucasians were sedentary." However, all are grouped as inactive. Similarly, Shephard (1967) compared $\dot{V}O_2$ max in groups described as "active" and "inactive." Active groups had higher $\dot{V}O_2$ max, except Scandinavians, whose values were similar (59 ml/kg/min). The higher values and the similarity of "active" and "inactive" groups in Scandinavians were regarded as arising from their more active lives compared to their counterparts in other areas. The description of "active" and "inactive" in Scandinavians seems inappropriate. Also, it is possible to quote several instances where $\dot{V}O_2$ max are similar, but physical activity might be expected to vary: e.g., young Norwegian lumberjacks (45 ml/kg/min) and Norwegian office workers (44 ml/kg/min) (Andersen 1966), Winnipeg furnace factory men (44 ml/kg/min) and office workers (44 ml/kg/min) (Cumming, 1967), nomadic Lapps (53 ml/kg/min) (Andersen, 1967a) and Stockholm males (52 ml/kg/min) (Åstrand, 1960).

Job titles are often poor indicators of activity. Indeed, the usefulness of activity description must be questioned. Because resting metabolism accounts for a large proportion of daily energy expenditure, perceived differences in daily exertion are associated with much smaller differences in daily energy expenditure. The difficulty of assessment of activity has been illustrated by Karvonen (1967). When subjects themselves made the assessment, those in moderate occupational activity had higher energy intakes (3,860 kcal/day) and, presumably, higher energy expenditures than those in light (3,240 kcal/day) or heavy (3,350 kcal/day) activity. However, when an interviewer made the classification, the light activity group had the highest energy intake and the heavy activity group had the lowest. Goldsmith and Hale (1971) investigated the relationship between habitual physical activity and physical fitness in United Kingdom policemen working in an office, as foot patrol men, or as car patrol men. There was no difference in fitness between the groups. Foot patrol officers had higher average heart rates at work (94± 4.4 versus 86± 5.7), but similar values in leisure time, although questionnaire results suggested that the time spent in active leisure pursuits in foot patrol officers was half that of the others (3.0 hr/week versus 6.5 hr/week).

Athletes and Heavy Occupations   The aerobic powers of athletes exceed those of the general population. The powers do vary according to event specificity, but the difference is always true for track athletes. Natural endowment is probably the important factor (Åstrand and Rodahl, 1970), so a consideration of activity and fitness in these groups may be confounded by genetic factors. This situation may also obtain when considering workers in heavy occupations. Mining, forestry work, and polar expeditions represent some extremes of physical activity (Durnin and Passmore, 1967). Some forestry workers have been found to have high aerobic capacities (Åstrand and Rodahl, 1970, but see Andersen, 1966). In a group of eight young Norwegian students who undertook a 10-week journey across the Arctic ice cap, a 10% decrease in $\dot{V}o_2$ max was found: 54 ml/kg/min to 48 ml/kg/min (Andersen, 1967b). The decrease in fitness with high levels of activity was unexpected.

RELATION OF ACTIVITY
PATTERNS TO LEVELS OF PHYSICAL FITNESS

A possible explanation for a lack of relationship between habitual physical activity and fitness could be that it is not mean daily energy expenditure levels that are important, but intensity of effort or peak levels. It is possible that a factory worker and a squash-playing bank clerk could have similar daily energy expenditures, yet entirely different activity patterns and aerobic powers. There is little disagreement that variations in fitness (aerobic power) of 10-20% can be brought about in an individual, the magnitude depending on the initial level of fitness of the subject and the intensity of effort.

Karvonen, Kentala, and Mustala (1957) found that a daily 30-min treadmill run for 4 weeks did not increase the working performance unless the heart rate exceeded 150 beats per min. However, Durnin, Brockway, and Whitcher (1960) observed increases in "fitness" in terms of pulmonary ventilation, oxygen extraction, oxygen consumption, and heart rate during a standardized treadmill test in young untrained men who walked 20 km daily over 2 weeks. Heart rates in the training sessions were 120−130/min. Shephard (1968) found no evidence for a training threshold in a sedentary North American population, but it was expected that in subjects of above average fitness a threshold would exist and that activity would have to be correspondingly more vigorous and intense to maintain or increase fitness: "Cardiorespiratory fitness is best improved by 20−30 min of vigorous exercise five times per week."

Are the peak activity levels in the groups of high fitness sufficient to cause or maintain their fitness? In laboratory tests of Igloolik Eskimos, cardiac frequencies of 120 and 150 beats/min were found at $\dot{V}_{O_2}$ of 1.8 and 2.5 liters/min (9−12.5 kcal/min) (Rode and Shephard, 1971). Only one of over 70 measurements or estimations of energy expenditure in daily activities exceeded 9 kcal/min/65 kg male (Godin and Shephard, 1973). Cardiac frequencies would undoubtedly exceed these levels in some of the other activities, but the total number of occasions does not seem high. If Eskimos are a trained group, work intensity and heart rate to maintain fitness would have to be higher than in the studies mentioned above.

In New Guineans, where heart rates of 110−120 beats/min are found with energy expenditures of 7.5 kcal/min, there are few activities involving energy expenditures greater than 7.5 kcal/min that are pursued for any length of time (Norgan, Ferro-Luzzi, and Durnin, 1974). This is also true of activities requiring 5.0−7.5 kcal/min. In Italian shipyard workers, 18% of active tasks were in this category. Thus, in contrast to the laboratory situation, it is difficult to see from this cursory analysis of field studies how a training effect would arise and be maintained.

Durnin (1967) has described activity patterns in subjects of different age, sex, body build, and occupation both at work and at leisure. Males in sedentary occupations spent 45 min/day in moderate activity (5.0−7.4 kcal/65 kg/min), 2 min/day in heavy activity (7.5−10.0 kcal/65 kg/min), and 2 min/day in very heavy activity (> 10 kcal/65kg/min). All but 8 min were spent in leisure. In moderate occupations, such as factory work, 67 min were spent in moderate activity; heavy workers, such as farmers, coal miners, and forestry workers spent 173 min in moderate activity, 21 min in heavy activity, and 3 min in very heavy activity. There were large intersubject differences. Workers in heavy occupations spent little time in intense activity and differed mainly in the amount of moderate activity they performed. They spent less time in activity at the three levels in their leisure time. However, 20 min/day of heavy activity (7.5−10.0 kcal/65 kg/min) could have a significant training effect. This level of activity when pursued for 15 min/day has been regarded as beneficial in preventing coronary heart disease (Morris et al., 1973). This more detailed analysis suggests that in heavy occupations (daily energy expenditures of 3,500 kcal/day and over, 54 kcal/kg/day) (Durnin and Passmore, 1967), peak activities are sufficient for a training effect to arise.

Activity in Childhood

So far fitness has been compared with contemporary activity. There is the suggestion that activity in childhood or adolescence may determine the potential for exercise in adult life (Åstrand and Rodahl, 1970), although this has been questioned (Weber, Kartodihardjo, and Klissouras, 1976). There is little that can be said about the childhood activity of the subjects in the studies that have been considered. The measurement of activity and energy expenditure in children is fraught with difficulties because of their characteristic pattern of behavior. One approach is to subtract the energy requirements for maintenance and growth from observed intakes (FAO/WHO, 1973). Cotes (1976) is of the opinion that measurement of the transfer factor of the lung enables the effect of short-term (recent) variations in activity to be separated from the combined effect of activity in childhood plus constitutional factors and the transfer factor may contribute additional information to that provided by exercise responses.

In contrast to activity, there is a fair amount of information on aerobic capacity in children (see Cumming, 1967). Igloolik Eskimo children have very high predicted aerobic capacities (Rode and Shephard, 1971). Lapp values are slightly less than those of Stockholm children, and both are higher than North American children. By the age of 16 years, there is little difference between Lapps and Winnipeg children. The role of activity in contributing to these differences is not obvious. The amount of physical education in Swedish educational institutions (Åstrand, 1967a) does not seem much different to those in other European countries, and work performance has been observed to fall during vacations (Åstrand, 1967b). Similarly, the higher aerobic powers in Scandinavian adults are regarded as real differences (Shephard, 1967), yet these have not been related to quantitative measures of activity.

NUTRITION

The level of nutrition is one of the environmental factors able to modify the ability to perform strenuous physical work (Åstrand, 1973). Acute deficiency of several vitamins, particularly those of the B group, or variations in the proportions of the proximate principle may elicit this effect (Christensen and Hansen, 1939; Bergström et al., 1967), but caloric undernutrition has been the subject of most investigation. The authoritative studies by Keys and colleagues showed a reduction in maximal performance capacity with experimentally-induced undernutrition (Keys et al., 1950). Undernutrition brings about a number of responses and adaptations, including a reduction in physical activity. This is well documented in the Minnesota study and in field situations (Keller and Kraut, 1962), so that it is difficult to separate the effects of undernutrition from physical activity. This holds true for the reverse situation. The reported increase in $\dot{V}O_2$ max in Bantu mine workers over the initial months of employment was accompanied by both an abundant, balanced diet (4,000 kcal/day) and regular moderate physical work (Wyndham et al., 1966). The observation that $\dot{V}O_2$ max in Bushmen decreased during a period of drought is interesting (Wyndham, 1967). Body weight was 8% lower after the 5-year period of drought, and $\dot{V}O_2$ max ml/kg/min fell 11%. Lee (1968) found that the food intakes of Bushmen during the third year of drought were adequate, but that neighboring groups of farmers were undernourished.

The effect of 3 years supplementation of poor diets on work output and aerobic power has been investigated in Guatemalan peons (Viteri, 1971). The supplemented group had higher daily energy expenditures: 3,450 kcal versus 2,700 kcal. The amount of work produced before exhaustion in laboratory tests was higher, although not significantly, but the $\dot{V}O_2$ max (42 ml/kg) was identical to that of a poorly nourished group, confounding the common understanding of the relationship between nutrition, activity, and fitness.

Overnutrition may arise by an increased energy intake or decreased utilization. Reduced physical activity has been implicated in the development of obesity. There is evidence that the obese are less active (Bullen, Reed, and Mayer, 1964), and in experimental overnutrition of young adult males the time spent in sedentary activities increased with weight gain (Norgan, unpublished).

Energy intake restriction with maintained or increased physical activity may be found in weight reduction of the obese. Maximal aerobic capacity in boys was observed to decrease both in absolute values and on the basis of fat-free mass (Šprynarova and Pařízková, 1965).

The $\dot{V}O_2$ max in obese Italian shipyard workers (31% fat) was the same as in normal subjects when expressed as ml/kg/FFM/min. The obese had similar energy expenditures and occupational categories. Others have reported that obesity imposes a severe limitation on physical work capacity (Dempsey et al., 1966; Davies et al., 1975).

In summary, the differential effects of nutrition and physical activity are difficult to separate in groups going about their everyday life.

Genetic Factors

If levels of habitual physical activity cannot be shown to have a clear association with fitness, then constitutional factors may explain the differences observed between individuals and groups. It is possible that successful communities in demanding habitats are composed of individuals selected for greater ability for prolonged or high levels of physical exertion. Similarly, the composition of groups engaged in heavy occupations may differ from the general population by self-selection. There is little doubt that successful athletes represent examples of high natural endowment for particular tasks. Genetic endowment for fitness has not proved amenable to investigation, and this may have resulted in undue emphasis on levels of habitual physical activity.

It has been suggested from studies on identical and nonidentical twins that 94% of the variation of maximum oxygen uptake is inherited (Klissouras, 1971; Klissouras, Pirnay, and Peti, 1973). Shephard (1976) regards this estimate as too high, because it is difficult to ensure that twins are exposed to the same environment, and he considers that in the extreme case genetic factors could account for 67% and training for 33%. Nevertheless, whatever the exact contribution is, if it is accepted that it varies within populations, it may be unreasonable to exclude variations between populations.

CONCLUSIONS

It is commonly assumed that physical fitness is related to physical activity. In groups with high physical fitness, such as New Guineans and Eskimos, habitual physical activity is not markedly greater than in many Western industrial workers. Similar levels of fitness have been found in groups with varying energy expenditures. The available information on peak levels of activity does not explain these apparent paradoxes. Genetic endowment is an accepted explanation for part of the superior performance in athletes, but this has not been invoked to explain differences between ethnic groups.

Assessment of habitual physical activity has proved difficult. Energy expenditures at work and in nonoccupational activities are required, and more data on peak rates should be collected. Information of this kind and fewer unwarranted assumptions may disclose more precisely the relative contribution of physical activity and genetic factors to fitness.

REFERENCES

Aghemo, P., Limas. F. P., and Sassi, G. 1971. Maximal aerobic power in primitive Indians. Int. Z. Angew. Physiol. 29: 337–342.

190   Norgan and Ferro-Luzzi

Andersen, K. L. 1966. Work capacity of selected populations. In P. T. Baker and J. S. Weiner (eds.), The Biology of Human Adaptability. Clarendon Press, Oxford.

Andersen, K. L. 1967a. Ethnic group differences in fitness for sustained and strenuous muscular exercise. Canad. Med. Assoc. J. 96(8): 32–38.

Andersen, K. L. 1967b. The effect of physical training with and without cold exposure upon physiological indices of fitness for work. Canad. Med. Assoc. J. 96: 801–803.

Andersen, K. L., Shephard, R. J., Denolin, H., Varnauskas, E., and Masironi, R. 1971. Fundamentals of Exercise Testing. WHO, Geneva.

Åstrand, I. 1960. Aerobic work capacity in men and women with special reference to age. Acta Physiol. Scand. 49 (suppl. 169).

Åstrand, P. O. 1967a. General Discussion in Nutrition and Physical Activity. Symp. Swed. Nutr. Found. V: 142.

Åstrand, P. O. 1967b. Concluding remarks, Symposium on Physical Activity and Cardiovascular Health. Canad. Med. Assoc. J. 96: 910.

Åstrand, P. O. 1973. Nutrition and physical performance. in M. Rechcigl (ed.), Food, Nutrition, and Health. World Rev. Nutr., Diet., 16: 59–79.

Åstrand, P. O., and Rodahl, K. 1970. In Textbook of Work Physiology. McGraw-Hill Book Company, New York.

Bergström, J., Hermansen, L., Hultman, E., and Saltin, B. 1967. Diet, muscle glycogen and physical performance. Acta Physiol. Scand. 71: 140–150.

Bullen, B. A., Reed, R. B., and Mayer, J. 1964. Physical activity of obese and non-obese adolescent girls. Appraisal by motion picture samples. Am. J. Clin. Nutr. 14: 211–223.

Christensen, E. H., and Hansen, O. 1939. Arbeitsfähigkeit und Ernähung. (Work capability and nutrition.) Skand. Arch. Physiol. 81: 160–189.

Clark, C., and Haswell, M. R. 1970. The Economics of Subsistence Agriculture. 4th ed. MacMillan, London.

Conklin, H. C. 1957. Hanunoo agriculture in the Philippines. F.A.O. Forestry Development Paper no. 12. FAO, Rome.

Cotes, J. E. 1976. Genetic and environmental determinants of the physiological response to exercise. Medicine and Sport, Vol 9, Advances in Exercise Physiology, 188–202. Karger, Basel.

Cotes, J. E., Anderson, H. R., and Patrick, J. M. 1974. Lung function and the response to exercise in New Guineans, role of genetic and environmental factors. Phil. Trans. R. Soc. Lond. B. 268: 349–361.

Cotes, J. E., Berry, G., Burkinshaw, L., Davies, C. T. M., Hall, A. M., Jones, P. R. M., and Knibbs, A. V. 1973a. Cardiac frequency during submaximal exercise in young adults; relation to lean body mass, total body potassium and amount of leg muscle. Q. J. Exp. Physiol. 58: 239–250.

Cotes, J. E., and Davies, C. T. M. 1969. Factors underlying the capacity for exercise: A study in physiological anthropometry. Proc. R. Soc. Med. 62: 620–624.

Cotes, J. E., Davies, C. T. M., Edholm, O. G., Healy, M. J. R., and Tanner, J. M. 1969. Factors relating to the aerobic capacity of 46 healthy British males and females, ages 18 to 28 years. Proc. R. Soc. Lond. B 174: 91–114.

Cotes, J. E., Hall, A. M., Johnson, G. R., Jones, P. R. M., and Knibbs, A. V. 1973b. Decline with age of cardiac frequency during submaximal exercise in healthy women. J. Physiol., (London) 238: 24–25.

Cumming, G. R. 1967. Current levels of fitness. Canad. Med. Assoc. J. 96: 868–877.

Davies, C. T. M. 1968. Limitations to the prediction of maximum oxygen intake from cardiac frequency measurements. J. Appl. Physiol. 24: 700–706.

Davies, C. T. M. 1973. Relationship of maximum power output to productivity and absenteeism of East African sugar cane workers. Br. J. Indust. Med. 30: 146–154.

Davies, C. T. M., Barnes, C., Fox, R. H., Ojikutu, R. O., and Samueloff, A. S. 1972. Ethnic differences in physical working capacity. J. Appl. Physiol. 33: 726–732.

Davies, C. T. M., Godfrey, S., Light, M., Sargeaunt, A. J., and Zeidifand, E. 1975. Cardiopulmonary response to exercise in obese girls and young women. J. Appl. Physiol. 38: 373–376.

Davies, C. T. M., Mbelwa, D., Crockford, G., and Weiner, J. S. 1973. Exercise tolerance and body composition of male and female Africans aged 18–30 years. Hum. Biol. 45: 31–40.

Dempsey, J. A., Reddan, J. A., Balke, B., and Rankin, J. 1966. Work capacity determinants and physiologic cost of weight supported work in obesity. J. Appl. Physiol. 1815–1820.

diPrampero, P. E., and Cerretelli, P. 1969. Maximal muscular power (aerobic and anaerobic) in African natives. Ergonomics 12: 51–59.

Durnin, J. V. G. A. 1967. Activity patterns in the community. Canad. Med. Assoc. J. 96: 882–886.

Durnin, J. V. G. A. 1975. Unsolved problems in establishing international standards for energy requirements. In A. Chavez, H. Bourges, and S. Basta (eds.), Proc. IX Intern. Congr. Nutr. 1: 35–42. Karger, Basel.

Durnin, J. V. G. A., and Brockway, J. M. 1959. Determination of the total daily energy expenditure in man by indirect calorimetry: Assessment of the accuracy of a modern technique. Br. J. Nutr. 13: 41–53.

Durnin, J. V. G. A., Brockway, J. M., and Whitcher, H. W. 1960. Effects of a short period of training of varying severity on some measurements of physical fitness. J. Appl. Physiol. 15: 161–165.

Durnin, J. V. G. A., and Passmore, R. 1967. Energy, Work and Leisure. Heinemann, London.

Durnin, J. V. G. A., and Rahaman, M. M. 1967. The assessment of the amount of fat in the human body from measurements of skinfold thickness. Br. J. Nutr. 21: 681–689.

Edholm, O. G. 1970. The changing pattern of human activity. Ergonomics 13: 625–643.

Edwards, R. H. T., Miller, G. J., Hearn, C. E. D., and Cotes, J. E. 1972. Pulmonary function and exercise responses in relation to body composition and ethnic origin in Trinidadian males. Proc. R. Soc. Lond. Br. 181: 407–420.

FAO/WHO. 1973. Energy and protein requirements. FAO Nutrition Meeting Report series no. 52, FAO, Rome.

Fidanza, F. 1974. Tabelle di composizione degli alimenti. (Table of composition of foodstuffs.) Idelson, Napoli.

Godin, G., and Shephard, R. J. 1973. Activity patterns of the Canadian Eskimo. In O. G. Edholm, and E. K. E. Gunnersun (eds.), Polar Human Biology. Heinemann, London.

Goldsmith, R., and Hale, T. 1971. Relationship between habitual physical activity and physical fitness. Am. J. Clin. Nutr. 24: 1489–1493.

Gorou, P. 1966. The Tropical World. 4th ed. Longman, London.

Harrison, G. A., and Walsh, R. J. 1974. A discussion on human adaptability in a tropical ecosystem: An I.B.P. human biological investigation of two New Guinea communities. Phil. Trans. Soc. Lond. Br. 268: 221–400.

Hipsley, E. H., and Kirk, N. E. 1965. Studies of dietary intake and the expenditure of energy by New Guineans. Technical Paper 147. South Pacific Commission, Noumea.

Karvonen, M. J. 1967. Nutrition in heavy manual labour. In Nutrition and Physical Activity, V Symp. Swedish Nutr. Found, pp. 59–63. Blix. G., Uppsala.

Karvonen, M. J., Kentala, E., and Mustala, O. 1957. The effects of training on heart rate. Ann. Med. Exp. Biol. Fenn. 35: 307–315.

Keller, and Kraut. 1962. Work and nutrition. World Rev. Nutr. Diet. 3: 67–81.

Keys, A. 1970. Physical activity and the epidemiology of coronary heart disease. In Physical Activity and Ageing, Medicine and Sport, Vol. 4., pp. 250–266. Karger, Basel.

Keys, A., Brozek, J., Henschel, A., Mickelsen, O., and Taylor, H. L. 1950. The Biology of Human Starvation, pp. 714–748. The University of Minnesota Press, Minneapolis.

Klissouras, V. 1971. Heritability of adaptive variation. J. Appl. Physiol. 31: 338–334.

Klissouras, V., Pirnay, F., Petit, J. M. 1973. Adaptation to maximal effort: Genetics and age. J. Appl. Physiol. 35: 288–293.

Lea, D. A. M. 1970. Activity studies in New Guinea villages. Papua-New Guinea Agric. J. 21: 118–126.

Lee, R. B. 1968. What hunters do for a living, or, how to make out on scarce resources. In R. B. Lee, and I. Devore (eds.), Man the Hunter, p 30. Aldine Publishing Company, Chicago.

Maksud, M. G., Spurr, G. B., and Barac-Nieto, M. 1976. The aerobic power of several groups of labourers in Columbia and the United States. Europ. J. Appl. Physiol. 35: 173–182.

McCarthy, F. D., and McArthur, M. 1960. The food quest time in Aboriginal economic life. In G. P. Mountford (ed.), Anthropology and Nutrition, 2 Melbourne University Press, Parkville.

Miller, G. J., Cotes, J. E., Hall, A. M., Salvosa, C. B., and Ashworth, A. 1972. Lung function and exercise performance of healthy Caribbean men and women of African ethnic origin. Q.J. Exp. Physiol. 57: 325–341.

Morris, J. N., Chave, S. P. W., Adam, C., Sirey, C., Epstein, L., and Sheehan, D. J. 1973. Vigorous exercise in leisure time and incidence of coronary heart disease. Lancet i: 333–339.

Norgan, N. G., Ferro-Luzzi, A., and Durnin, J. V. G. A. 1974. The energy and nutrient intake and the energy expenditure of 204 New Guinean adults. Phil. Trans. R. Soc. Lond. Br. 268: 309–348.

Payne, P. R. 1975. Safe protein-calorie ratios in diets. The relative importance of protein and energy intake as causal factors in malnutrition. Am. J. Clin. Nutr. 28: 281–286.

Pugh, L. G. C. 1966. A programme for physiological studies of high altitude peoples. In P. T. Baker, and J. S. Weiner (eds.), The Biology of Human Adaptability, pp. 521–532. Clarendon, Oxford.

Rahn, H., Fenn, W. O., and Otis, A. B. 1949. Daily variations of vital capacity, residual air and expiratory reserve including a study of the residual air method. J. Appl. Physiol. 1: 725–736.

Rappaport, R. A. 1967. Pigs for the Ancestors. Yale University Press, New York.

Rode, A., and Shephard, R. J. 1971. Cardiorespiratory fitness of an Arctic community. J. Appl. Physiol. 31: 519–526.

Sahlins, M. 1974. Stone Age Economics. Tavistock, London.

Schaefer, O. 1971. When the Eskimo comes to town. Nutr. Today 6: 6−8.

Scudder, T. 1971. Gathering among African woodland savannah cultivators. Zambian Paper, no. 5.

Shephard, R. J. 1967. Commentary in Proc. Internat. Symp. Physical Activity and Cardiovascular Health. Canad. Med. Assoc. J. 96: 878.

Shephard, R. J. 1968. Intensity, duration and frequency of exercise as determinants of the response to a training regime. Int. Z. Angew. Physiol. 26: 272−278.

Shephard, R. J. 1974. Work physiology and activity patterns of circumpolar Eskimos and Ainu. Hum. Biol. 46: 263−294.

Shephard, R. J. 1976. Cardio-respiratory fitness. A new look at maximum oxygen intake. Medicine and Sport, Vol. 9, Advances in Exercise Physiology, pp. 61−84. Karger, Basel.

Shephard, R. J., Allen, C., Benade, A. J. S., Davies, C. T. M., Di Prampero, P. E., Hedman, R., Merriman, J. E., Myhre, K., and Simmons, R. 1968a. The maximum oxygen intake. An international reference standard of cardiorespiratory fitness. Bull. Wld. Hlth. Org. 38: 757−764.

Shephard, R. J., Allen, C., Benade, A. J. S., Davies, C. T. M., Di Prampero, P. E., Hedman, R., Merriman, J. E., Myhre, K., and Simmons, R. 1968b. Standardisation of submaximal exercise tests. Bull. World Health Org. 38: 765−775.

Shephard, R. J., and Rode, A. 1973. Fitness for arctic life: The cardiorespiratory status of the Canadian Eskimo. In O. G. Edholm and E. Gunnerson (eds.), Polar Human Biology. Heinemann, London.

Sinclair, H. M. 1953. The diet of Canadian Indians and Eskimos. Proc. Nutr. Soc. 12: 69−82.

Siri, W. E. 1956. The gross composition of the body. Advances in Biology and Medical Physiology, Vol. 4, pp. 239−280.

Spurr, G. B., Barac-Nieto, M., and Maksud, M. G. 1975. Energy expenditure cutting sugar cane. J. Appl. Physiol. 34: 990−996.

Šprynarova, S., and Pařízková, J. 1965. Changes in the aerobic capacity and body composition in obese boys after reduction. J. Appl. Physiol. 20: 934−937.

Viteri, F. E. 1971. Considerations of the effect of nutrition on the body composition and physical working capacity of young Guatemalan adults. In N. S. Scrimshaw, and A. M. Altschul (eds.), Amino-Acid Fortification of Protein Foods, pp. 350−375. M.I.T. Press, Cambridge.

Viteri, F. E., Torun, B., Galicia, J. C., and Herrera, E. 1971. Determining energy costs of agricultural activities by respirometer and energy balance techniques. Am. J. Clin. Nutr. 24: 1418−1430.

Weber, G., Kartodihardjo, W., and Klissouras, V. 1976. Growth and physical training with reference to heredity. J. Appl. Physiol. 40: 211−215.

Weiner, J. S., and Lourie, J. A. 1969. Human Biology. A guide to field methods. IBP Handbook No. 9. Blackwell, Oxford.

Woodburn, J. 1968. An introduction to Hazda ecology. In R. B. Lee, and I. de Vore (eds.), Man the Hunter. Aldine, Chicago.

Wyndham, C. H. 1967. Commentary. Canad. Med. Assoc. J. 96: 835.

Wyndham, C. H., Strydom, N. B., Leary, W. P., Williams, C. G., and Morrison, J. F. 1966. Studies of the maximum capacity of men for physical effort. Part III. The effects on the maximum oxygen intake of young males of a regime of regular exercise and an adequate diet. Int. Z. Angew. Physiol. 22: 304−310.

Interrelationships Between Nutrition, Physical Activity, and Physical Fitness

S. Suzuki, S. Oshima, E. Tsuji, K. Tsuji, F. Ohta

Rapid industrialization and economic development have greatly affected the living conditions of the Japanese population. The new living conditions in turn have remarkably influenced the physical fitness of the nation. The first part of this chapter includes some aspects of physical fitness of the whole nation in recent years, and suggests a close relationship between nutrition and physical activity. The second part explores, through a brief report on a series of animal experiments, the causal interrelationships among nutrition, physical activity, and physical fitness. Finally, in the third part, the results of a recent extensive survey are presented which suggest that the past concept of energy requirements for Japanese people must be changed.

SURVEYS ON THE PHYSICAL FITNESS OF THE JAPANESE POPULATION

Chronological Variations of the Whole Population: Nutrient Intake

Individual average intakes per day since 1950, quoted from the nutritional survey conducted by the Ministry of Health and Welfare, are shown in Figure 1. During the past 22 years, the total energy intake has increased no more than a few percent. The highest increase rates are seen in fats and animals protein. Fat and oil intake has increased three times, reaching a level of 50 g. This amount is not high when compared with the consumption in some foreign countries, however. One problem related to the greater fat and oil consumption is a remarkable increase of animal fats intake. Although the ratio of animal fats to total fats and oils was only one-third in the past, it is more than 50% at

Chronological Change of Nutritive Intake
(The Whole Nation)

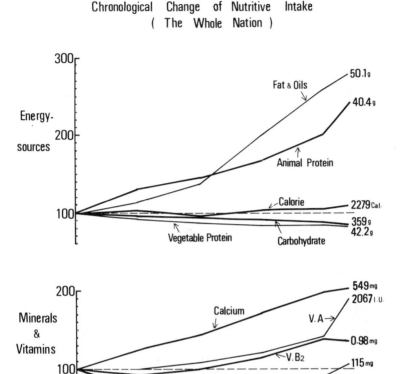

Figure 1. Individual average intakes per day from 1950–1972 (from Ministry of Health and Welfare, 1975). Fats and animal protein show highest increase rates.

present. Animal protein has also increased to over one-half of the total protein. On the contrary, carbohydrate and vegetable protein have decreased. With regard to minerals and vitamins, calcium and vitamin A have increased greatly, but vitamin B_1, B_2, and C have remained about the same.

Physical Activity   The most useful information in understanding the trend of physical activity in the whole nation is the distribution of the population classified by work intensity, which is estimated from the census and data provided by the Committee of Energy Requirements in Japan (Table 1) (Ministry of Health and Welfare, 1975). In 1960, the population of the moderate activity group was the largest, but it has sharply decreased since 1965. Most of the population moved to the

Table 1. Population distribution by activity

Work group	Sex	Energy expenditure (cal/day)	Percentage of population			
			1960	1965	1970	1980
Very light	M	2,300	17	22	25	30
	F	1,800				
Light	M	2,500	35	39	41	43
	F	2,000				
Moderate	M	3,000	46	38	33	27
	F	2,400				
Heavy	M	3,500	1	1	1	0
	F	2,800				
			100	100	100	100

light activity group, and simultaneously the population of the very light activity group rapidly increased. The very heavy activity group (4,000 kcal for males) had already disappeared 10 years ago. There are some exceptional cases in the heavy class at present, but they will no doubt disappear within 5 years or so.

Body Size   The average height of the Japanese had increased by 1 cm per decade until World War II, but began greatly decreasing as a result of the war—especially the height of young people, which declined to the level recorded in 1900. However, the recovery of height was remarkable after the war. Postwar growth rate was several times more rapid than the growth rate before the war. Figure 2 shows that there are signs of a slowing down in adolescent boys, although no sign of slowing down can be seen in girls.

Function   The only nationwide survey on the physiological functions that exists is the annual report of performance tests that the Ministry of Education started 10 years ago. Therefore, one can only evaluate this factor over a limited period. Various functions such as side-step, grip strength, vertical jump, bending forward, step-test, 50-m dash, broad jump, handball throwing, and chinning have all improved. However, back strength (Figure 3) and endurance running (Figure 4) did not always improve (Ministry of Education, 1974).

Death Rates   Although death rates of infectious diseases such as lung tuberculosis and pneumonia decreased sharply, those of cerebral embolism and ischemic heart disease have been increasing, and are as much as two or three times higher than 10 years ago. The death rates for diabetes, malignant neoplasms, and liver cirrhosis have been increasing. On the other hand, the death rate for cerebral hemorrhage, which had

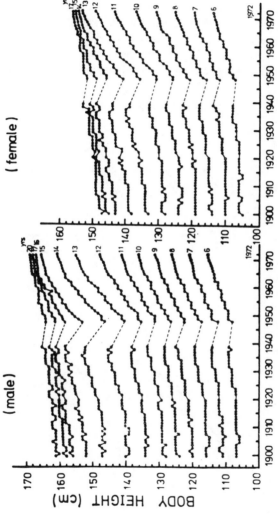

Figure 2. Pre- and postwar acceleration rate of body height. There was a regression during World War II, but growth rate picked up again after the war.

been highest in Japan, has been decreasing over the past 10 years. These trends are presumed to be closely related to nutrition and physical activity.

Urban and Rural: Nutrition and Physical Activity

Rural people in Japan had generally consumed excessive amounts of starchy food, and consequently, their intake of other nutrients were insufficient. However, as their income increased in recent years, their diet has improved gradually (Ministry of Health and Welfare, 1974). For a long time, agricultural labor had been typical heavy labor in Japan, but it has changed to moderate labor because of mechanization.

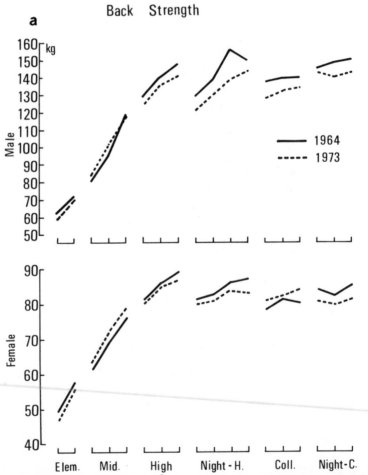

Figure 3. Nationwide comparison of back strength (a) and endurance running (b) in Japanese males and females between 1964 and 1973. From Ministry of Education, 1974.

On the other hand, activity of the urban people also moved from light to very light labor because of severe lack of physical activity. Therefore, the physical activity level of the rural population is still higher by two grades than that of the urban population.

Body Size   Rural people apparently have a smaller body size than the urban. The average height and weight of rural people is lower than that of the urban. In chest circumference, however, which is proportional to physical activity, the rural are superior to the urban (Ministry of Education, 1974).

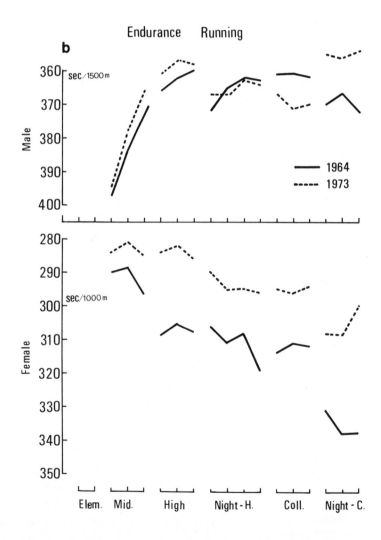

Function   With the exceptions of tests of strength (Figure 4a) and speedy walking (Figure 4b), the rural people are inferior in performance to the urban (Ministry of Education, 1974). It may be assumed that the rural inhabitants are not suitable for these kinds of sportlike performance tests because their agricultural labor consists more of static muscular work, i.e., they are not speedy and dynamic, and hold peculiar posture, etc. However, Figures 5a and b show clearly the reason for this result (Tamura, 1975). Although the maximal oxygen uptake of the rural people is superior, they do not perform as well on the 5-min running test as those living in urban areas.

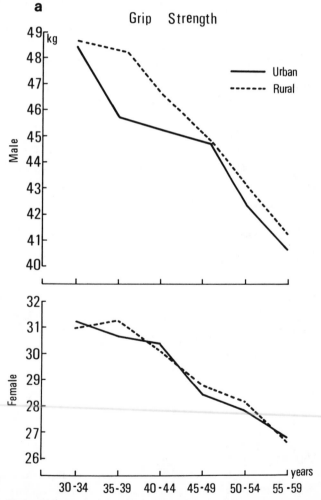

Figure 4. Nationwide comparison of grip strength (a) and fast walking (b) in rural and urban males and females.

CAUSAL RELATIONSHIPS IN ANIMALS
BETWEEN BODY SIZE AND INTERNAL ORGANS

Influence of Nutrition and Physical Activity

Male rats of the Wistar strain, 5-weeks-old and weighing approximately 65 g, were used. The animals were assigned at random to four experimental groups, each consisting of 18 rats. Two groups were fed ad libitum a high carbohydrate diet simulating the Japanese rural diet, and the remaining two groups were fed a high protein-high fat diet as found in Western countries (Table 2) (Suzuki et al., 1968). One subgroup

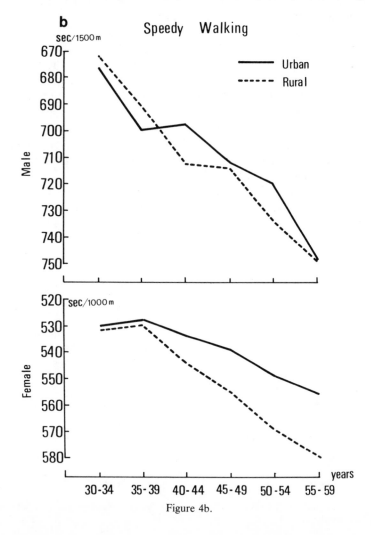

Figure 4b.

from each of the two dietary groups was kept in an individual cage equipped with a revolving wheel, 1 m in circumference and 8 cm in width, which could be used voluntarily. The revolution count was recorded daily.

The highest weight gain was found in the high protein-high fat diet nonexercising group, and the lowest gain in the high carbohydrate exercised group. Although a high protein-high fat diet always promoted weight gain in the animals, physical exercise resulted in the retardation of weight gain, as was observed when comparing the exercised and nonexercised animals of each dietary group. These trends can be observed also in the growth curves of the tail and the body length, although differences were not so great as in the weight gains.

In the internal organs, the nonexercising group had twice as much adipose tissue as the exercising group and less developed muscle per unit body weight (Table 3). The cholesterol content of the aorta was found to be higher in the high protein—high fat dietary group than in the high carbohydrate group, but the serum cholesterol concentration showed a reverse relation (Table 4). The fat used in all diets was soybean oil only, but the nature of fat will have to be taken into consideration in further experiments. The physical exercise imposed during the long period may decrease the cholesterol concentration of both aorta and serum, irrespective of the diets.

The diets caused distinct differences in the weight and length of the femora, i.e., there were heavier weights and longer lengths in the

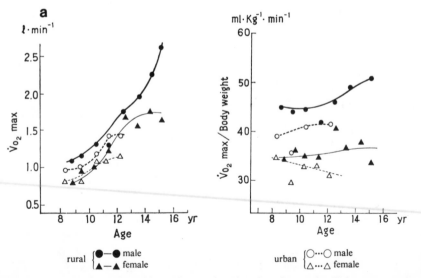

Figure 5. Comparison of aerobic work capacity (a) and work capacity (b) between rural and urban adolescents.

high protein-high fat dietary group than in the high carbohydrate group. No significant differences, however, could be found between the exercised and the nonexercised animals, although the former seemed to be inferior. Ash and calcium contents of the femora in each group were both apparently higher in the high protein-high fat groups than in the high carbohydrate ones. The high protein-high fat dietary

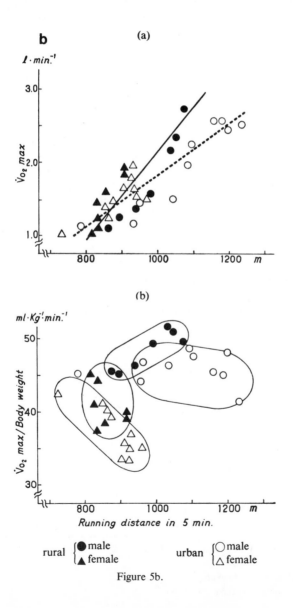

Figure 5b.

Table 2.   Diet composition

	High carbohydrate diet		High protein-high fat diet	
	Weight %	Cal %	Weight %	Cal %
Dextrin	75.0	76.7	45.0	39.8
Casein	9.7	9.9	23.0	20.3
Soybean oil	5.0	11.5	19.0	37.8
Yeast	4.0		5.0	
Liber oil	0.3		0.4	
Fiber	2.0		2.6	
Salt mixture	4.0		5.0	
Cal/100 g	391.0		453.0	

Vitamin B_1, B_2, Cholin supplemented, and E supplemented.
From Suzuki et al., 1968.

group had a significantly higher amount of ash and calcium in the nonexercised than in the exercised animals.

From these results, the following conclusions can be drawn. Quantitative and qualitative development of the bone are influenced only by nutrition and not by physical exercise. Size and weight of the bone of animals fed the high protein-high fat diet were far superior to those fed the high carbohydrate diet. Physical exercise did not promote the size and weight of the bone at all. In both ash and calcium contents of the bone, a very similar tendency was observed in size and weight. As far as the influence of physical exercise on the mineral content is con-

Table 3.   Nutrition, physical exercise, and growth in groups of 18 rats

		High carbohydrate diet		High protein-high fat diet	
		Nonexercise	Exercise	Nonexercise	Exercise
Body weight	(g)	264.0	250.0	379.0[a]	296.0[b]
Body length	(cm)	22.1	22.2	24.4[a]	23.3[b]
Tail length	(cm)	17.1	16.8	18.3[a]	17.7[b]
Carcass	(g)	204.0	192.0	293.0[a]	232.0[b]
Fat deposit	(g)	6.44[c]	3.63	11.54[a]	4.67
(peri-renal)		(2.4)[d]	(1.3)[d]	(3.0)[d]	(1.6)[d]
Muscles (leg)	(g)	1.40	1.44	1.73[b]	1.72[b]
		(0.53)[d]	(0.58)[d]	(0.46)[d]	(0.58)[d]

[a] $p < 0.01$ between both diets and between nonexercise and exercise.
[b] $p < 0.01$ between both diets.
[c] $p < 0.01$ between nonexercise and exercise.
[d] Per body weight, percent.

Table 4. Nutrition, physical exercise, and growth in groups of 18 rats

		High carbohydrate diet		High protein-high fat diet	
		Nonexercise	Exercise	Nonexercise	Exercise
Heart	(g)	0.85	0.83	1.11[a]	1.01[b]
		(0.32)[c]	(0.33)[c]	(0.29)[c]	(0.34)[c]
Aorta	(mg)	53.7	54.2	60.5	54.2
		(0.020)[c]	(0.022)[c]	(0.016)[c]	(0.018)[c]
Cholesterol (aorta)	(mg/g)	1.51	1.47	1.60	1.58
Cholesterol (serum)	(mg/dl)	67	62	61	57

[a] $p < 0.01$ between both diets and between nonexercise and exercise.
[b] $p < 0.01$ between both diets.
[c] Per body weight, percent.

cerned, an undesirable effect was found during the developmental stage of the bone.

Of both nutrition and physical exercise, the latter seemed to be a more important and primary factor for the prevention of excessive fatness. This is because the nonexercised group had double the amount of adipose tissue in spite of its lower food intake.

Amount of Voluntary Exercise, Diet, Growth, and Survival Rate

A total of 100 male Wistar strain rats, 40-days-old and weighing 100−130 g at the time of the experiment, were randomly divided into four groups. Two groups were fed ad libitum a high carbohydrate diet simulating the Japanese rural diet, and the remaining two groups were fed a high protein-high fat Western type diet (Table 5). One subgroup of each of the two dietary groups was kept in an individual cage equipped with a voluntary-use revolving wheel. Daily running distance of the animals increased steadily during the first 100 days after birth, amounting to 2,200 m/day, on the average. This maximum level was maintained for 50 days, but thereafter it decreased rapidly at first and then gradually until finally it reached a constant and low level, 300 days after birth. The 100−150 day age range is the most active period in the rat, and corresponds roughly to the age of 11−14 years in man, if the growth curves of both species are compared. Many sociological factors, such as education and occupation, affect man's physiological status, but normally his highest level of physical activity is during adolescence.

As to the relationship between physical exercise and dietary composition, it was found that the quantitative curve of physical exercise of

Table 5.   Diet composition

	High carbohydrate diet		High protein-high fat diet	
	Weight %	Cal %	Weight %	Cal %
Dextrin	73.0	72.5	48.0	41.5
Casein	12.0	11.9	25.0	21.6
Soybean oil	3.0		4.0	
Lard	3.0	15.6	14.0	36.9
Vegetable oil g/100g	1.0		1.0	
Liver oil	0.3		0.3	
Vitamin mixture	0.85		0.85	
Choline chloride	0.15		0.15	
Salt mixture	4.0		4.0	
Fiber	2.7		2.7	
Cal/100g	403.0		463.0	

the group on the high protein-high fat diet always preceded the curve of the group on the high carbohydrate diet. That is, the former reached the maximum level and thereafter declined more quickly than the latter. The constant amount of physical exercise in the mature period was almost double in the high protein-high fat diet group in comparison with the high carbohydrate diet group. Therefore, it seems that a high protein-high fat diet accelerated growth and physical exercise during the period of development, and made the animal more active during the period of maturity, although mature animals fed a high protein-high fat diet were much larger in body size than the group fed the high carbohydrate diet.

Physical Exercise, Dietary Intake, and Growth   The caloric intakes of the high protein-high fat diet groups exceeded those of the high carbohydrate diet groups by almost 10%, corresponding to better growth in the former. In studying dietary intake in relation to physical exercise, the exercising animals consumed nearly 30% more than the nonexercising groups during the most active period (around the 140th day after birth), and 10% more in the later and less active period (around the 280th day after birth). Thus, physical exercise evidently promoted the dietary intake of the animals, but did not promote growth in body weight and length, retarding it instead.

Among the exercising animals, individual differences were observed in activity, dietary intake, and growth. To determine the interrelationships among these variables, the animals that exercised were divided into three groups according to the distance they ran: that is, less than 100 m, between 100 and 1,000 m, and more than 1,000 m per day. It was found that the more active the animals were, the greater amount of food they consumed and the smaller their growth was. This relationship was more pronounced when the amount of dietary intake was expressed per unit of body weight.

Survival Rate   The group that exercised on the high protein-high fat diet showed the highest survival rate, and the nonexercising group on the high protein-high fat diet presented the lowest. The rates of the high carbohydrate groups were mid-range between the two. Although this result must be confirmed in repeated studies, it is noteworthy that the high protein-high fat diet with physical exercise was found to improve the survival rate, but lack of physical exercise caused it to decrease. Many authors (McCay et al., 1939; Berg and Simms, 1961; Ross, 1961) have reported that restricted dietary intake or a low protein diet improved the survival rate, but limited proper growth. This was not so with the animals undergoing physical exercise.

Blood Pressure and Physical Exercise   Five-week-old male, spontaneously hypertensive rats (SHR) were divided into two groups, each consisting of 19 rats. Both groups were fed ad libitum a commercial diet for 24 weeks. One group was kept in individual cages equipped with a voluntarily revolving wheel, 1 m in circumference, as described earlier, and another group was kept in cages without the exercise wheel. In the second experiment, at the age of 11 weeks, their blood pressure rose to 180 mm Hg. The SHRs were divided into two groups, as in the first experiment, in order to observe whether voluntary exercise could have an influence even after SHRs distinctly grew hypertensive. In the third experiment, in order to clarify whether forced exercise gives the same results as voluntary exercise, one group of SHR was put into a specially designed apparatus consisting of a wire gauze cylinder revolving drum that was rotated by an electric motor, and the SHRs were compelled to walk for 5 hr a distance of 2,000 m every day. Blood pressure was measured by tail plethysmography and a blood sample was taken from the tail tip (50 μl).

Running distance of the exercised group amounted to 7,000 m/day on the average during the peak period of 11 weeks of age, which was about three times more than that of the normal Wistar strain rats. Growth rates of both groups were almost identical.

Blood pressure of the nonexercised group reached 200 mm Hg on the average at the age of 15 weeks. On the other hand, the value of the exercised group remained at 170 mm Hg (Figure 6a). Observation of the individual differences among the exercised animals demonstrated the following interrelationships: the more active the animals were, the lower their blood pressure (Figure 6b).

Plasma cholesterol concentrations of the exercised animals were always significantly lower than those of the nonexercised animals.

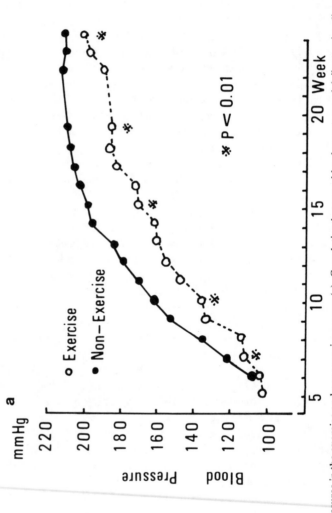

Figure 6. Blood pressures in the exercise and nonexercise groups (a). Correlation between blood pressure and daily running distance at 10, 15, 19, and 24 weeks of age (b). The more active animals had lower blood pressure.

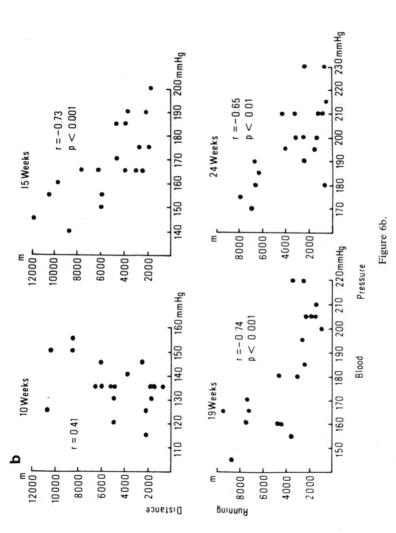

Figure 6b.

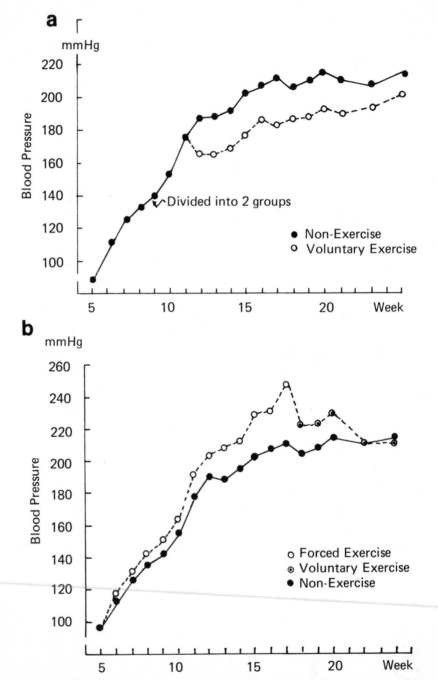

Figure 7. Blood pressures in nonexercise and voluntary exercise groups (a) and in forced, voluntary, and nonvoluntary exercise groups (b). Forced exercise is shown to increase blood pressure.

Exercise Begun in the Mature Period   In the second experiment, the SHRs began to run immediately after they were put in the cages equipped with the exercise wheels, and their running distance amounted to an average of 8,000 m/day after a few weeks. At the same time their blood pressure decreased from 180 mm Hg to 160 mm Hg. The blood pressure of the group without physical exercise increased from 180 mm Hg to 190 mm Hg during the same period (Figure 7a).

In the 3rd experiment, it was proved that forced exercise did not decrease the blood pressure at all, but increased it. Right after physical exercise was changed from forced to voluntary, blood pressure began to decrease (Figure 7b), in spite of almost the same running distance in both cases (Suzuki et al., 1968). Forced exercise was carried out every night in order to discover whether their day-night rhythm might be disturbed and thus increase the blood pressure (the forced exercise described above was conducted in the daytime for the authors' convenience). The effect of the forced exercise on the blood pressure was not changed by the nighttime exercise.

A NEW CONCEPT OF ENERGY
REQUIREMENTS FOR JAPANESE PEOPLE

The nutritional allowances for the Japanese (Ministry of Health and Welfare, 1974) have been revised every five years. Modifications are based on changes in body size, basal metabolism, activities, and new knowledge. Requirements are defined with regard to the energy expenditure in daily life. Recently, remarkable inactivity of the nation has distinctly decreased energy expenditure, resulting in undesirable influences upon physical fitness. Therefore, the past concept must now be reconsidered. How much physical exercise is necessary to keep healthy and to maintain enough physical ability for daily work? The minimum amount required to prevent obesity and various diseases common in adulthood should correspond to the energy requirements, and an additional amount leaving a margin to perform daily work without fatigue should correspond to the recommended energy allowances.

For such a purpose, the National Physical Fitness Research Team of Tsukuba University has carried out a wide and precise investigation on physical fitness of 1,356 inhabitants in Ibaraki Prefecture, age 20 to 80 years. Among subjective symptoms, the most frequently encountered was low back pain (nearly 50%), followed by fatigue, shoulder discomfort, gastric complaint, and breathlessness after physical effort in nearly 30% of the subjects. Moreover, these symptoms were widely distributed, without regard to sex, age, or profession, manifesting insufficient physical fitness. As to physical exercise, the subjects were engaged in walking, ramble, and calisthenics for the most part, and sports or running for only 1−2% of the time. Estimated amounts of exercise averaged 30 kcal/day for males and 15 kcal/day for females. An expenditure of more than 200 kcal/day was recorded at 15% in males and 10% in females.

In reference to the relationship between the amount of daily exercise and physical fitness tests, the greater the amount of exercise, the less frequent were both glycosuria and abnormal ECG (Figures 8a and b). Aging processes estimated from several kinds of performance tests indicated that males exercising more than 200 kcal/day and females more than 150 kcal/day seemed to be distinctly younger when compared with their chronological age, or with others who do not engage in any physical exercise in their daily life.

High frequency of the subjective symptoms such as low back pain, fatigue, etc. suggests that there is no margin left in their physical fitness for their daily life. To develop such a margin, positive training is necessary to promote their endurance ability and whole aerobic capacity of the organism. A standardized training program has been established by the Project Team of Exercise Prescription at the Research Centre of Physical Education (1976). During several years the Project Team, which consisted of researchers from more than 20 universities, conducted a series of careful studies of the relations between intensity, time per day, frequency per week, and kinds and periods of exercises. A guide called *Training Program for Health Promotion* was published. Based on further research and surveys in this field, it may be possible in the near future to decide on the exercise requirements and exercise allowances that should be equivalent to the energy requirements and caloric allowances for Japanese people. In the past, most research on energy metabolism has concentrated exclusively on energy efficiency: how energy consumption can be minimized in the field of humans as well as in animals, plants, etc. At present, however, the direction of the research should be directed toward improving health and promoting physical fitness, first of all in industrially developed countries.

Conclusions

Summarizing the results obtained from the statistical data and experimental measurements in research animals as well as in human subjects, it can be concluded that the physical fitness of the Japanese population during the past 20 years has been rapidly changing both in positive and negative directions. This is mainly because of the changes in nutrition and physical activity level, as observed in other countries with developing industrial production. Accordingly, the Nutritional Allowances Committee recommended not only nutritional improvements, but also an increase in daily physical exercise. For instance, physical

a

ECG vs Occupation   ECG vs Total Energy Expenditure

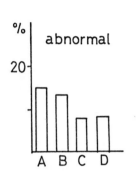

A: inactive sedent.
B: active sedent.
C: moderate
D: hard

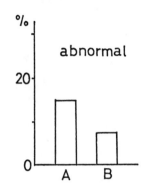

A: ~ 2,400 Cal

B: 2,400 Cal ~

b   Rate of positive glucosuria in each exercise group

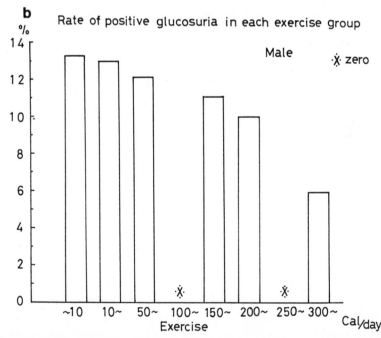

Figure 8. ECG compared to occupation and energy expenditure (a), and rate of positive glucosuria in each exercise group (b). The greater the amount of exercise, the less frequent were both glucosuria and abnormal ECG.

exercise corresponding to 200 kcal/day for sedentary men and house-wives are suggested, although the requirements and allowances of physical exercise are as yet not scientifically established.

REFERENCES

Berg, N. B., and Simms, H. S. 1961. Nutrition and longevity in the rat. J. Nutr. 74: 23–32.

MacCay, C. M., Ellis, G. H., Barnes, L. L., Smith, C. A. H., and Sperling, G. 1939. Chemical and pathological changes in aging and after retarded growth. J. Nutr. 18: 15–25.

Ministry of Education. 1973. Statistics of school health, pp. 32–39. Tokyo.

Ministry of Education. 1974. Survey of physical fitness, pp. 43–49. Tokyo.

Ministry of Health and Welfare. 1974. Present status of national nutrition, p. 211. Tokyo.

Ministry of Health and Welfare. 1975a. Nutritional allowances for Japanese. Tokyo.

Ministry of Health and Welfare. 1975b. Vital statistics. Tokyo.

National Physical Fitness Research Team of Tsukuba University. 1976. Studies on physical fitness and health of Japanese population, pp. 17–177. Tsukuba University, Ibaraki.

Research Center in Physical Education. 1976. Training program for health promotion, pp. 49–78. Kodansha, Tokyo.

Ross, M. H. 1961. Length of life and nutrition in the rat. J. Nutr. 75: 197–210.

Suzuki, S., Ohta, F., Tsuji, K., Oshima, S., Tsuji, E., Ohta, H., and Suzuki, H. 1968. Experimental studies on the interrelationships of nutrition, physical exercise and health components. Report 2. Influence on bone developments. Annual Report of National Institute of Nutrition, pp. 3–18. Tokyo.

Suzuki, S., Oshima, S., Ohta, F., Tsuji, K., Tsuji, E., and Mitsuishi, R. 1969. Experimental studies on the interrelationships of nutrition, physical exercise and health components. Report 3, Amount of physical exercise, dietary composition, growth and survival rate. Annual Report of National Institute of Nutrition, pp. 3–10. Tokyo.

Suzuki, S., and Oshima, S. 1976. Influence of physical exercise on blood pressure using the spontaneously hypertensive rat. Japan. J. Nutr. 34: 109–114.

Tamura, Y. 1975. Physical fitness of rural adolescents. Japan. Int. Progr. 4: 50–61.

Nutritional Status, Body Physique, and Work Output

K. Satyanarayana, A. Nadamuni Naidu, B. Chatterjee, B. S. Narasinga Rao

There have been several attempts in the past to determine the effects of malnutrition on work efficiency and work output (FAO, 1962; Bhavani, 1966; Satyanarayana et al., 1972). Although malnutrition has been shown to result in a reduction in maximal work capacity (Viteri, 1974), its effect, if any, on work output at submaximal work levels under normal work situations has not been clearly demonstrated in any direct study. Available information on the relationship between nutrition, on the one hand, and work output, on the other, relates largely to epidemiological studies (Keller and Kraut, 1962). Attempts in the past to directly relate malnutrition and work output have not been successful, primarily because of methodological difficulties (Bhavani, 1966; Satyanarayana et al., 1972). The present study is an attempt to quantify work output and relate it to the nutritional status of the workers.

Fifty-seven male workers in a local industry (IDL Chemicals Ltd., Hyderabad) were selected for this study. Their ages ranged from 20 to 35 years. Relevant details of the subjects are given in Table 1.

The industry chosen for the study provided all the amenities for the workers and a highly satisfactory working environment. The workers were provided with transportation to and from their residences. They received adequate medical care, and were also given an adequate meal in the middle of the working shift. The meal provided about half the day's requirements of calories and protein, i.e., 1,240 kcal and 25 g protein.

The job consisted of preparing safety fusewire for detonators, and represented a moderate level of physical activity. The job required the worker to stand at a place and carry out the following operations: pulling a wire, winding it around a metal bar and cutting it to a specified

The material contained in this chapter is reproduced from the *American Journal of Clinical Nutrition* 30:322, copyright 1977, by permission.

Table 1. Characteristics of the subjects (mean ± SD)

Anthropometrical factors		Social factors		Biochemical variables	
Height (cm)	163.5 ± 5.96	Age (years)	25.0 ± 3.3	Hemoglobin	15.9 ± 1.49
Weight (kg)	51.8 ± 5.74	Service (months)	25.9 ± 18.3	(g/100 ml)	
Body fat (%)	9.6 ± 2.12	Family size (total no.)	7.9 ± 3.5	Serum albumin	4.1 ± 0.45
				(g/100 ml)	
Lean body weight	46.7 ± 4.62	Family income	78.5 ± 30.9		
(fat-free weight, kg)		(Rs. per capita/month)			

length by means of a leg-operated machine. Twenty-five pieces of such wire were made into a bundle. Work output during an 8-hr shift was measured in terms of number of bundles produced, and could, therefore, be precisely quantified. The workers were given incentive pay according to the number of bundles produced, after fulfilling a minimum output of 90 bundles per day to earn their basic wages. There were three 8-hr shifts in a day, and the workers were assigned to all three shifts in a rotational sequence. Daily work output was recorded for each worker over a period of 3 months. Follow-up data were available on 46 workers.

The rate of work output was measured in all these workers in an 8-hr shift on four separate days by recording the number of bundles produced every 2 hr.

The nutritional status of the workers was assessed by clinical examination and anthropometry. Height, weight, and skinfold thicknesses were measured at the beginning of the study. From these anthropometric data, lean body weight (fat-free weight) was computed using formulas given by Pascale as adopted by other workers (Damon and Goldman, 1964) for body density and by Siri (1956) for percentage of fat. Hemoglobin and serum albumin were also measured at the beginning of the study. Information on the socioeconomic factors that may be expected to have influenced work output was also collected. Thus, data on marital status, family size, family income, work experience, and indebtedness were collected for each worker under study.

The anthropometric data, biochemical parameters, and other particulars of the workers studied are given in Table 1. The work output measured in terms of bundles produced by workers in different body weight groups is given in Table 2.

Biochemical tests and clinical examinations indicated that the subjects were not suffering from any overt nutritional deficiency. Anthropometric data, however, suggested widely different nutritional backgrounds. The body weights of the workers were recorded every month and all of them maintained their body weight within 1 kg. There

Table 2. Relationships between body weight and productivity and other variables

Body weight (kg)	N	Production[a] (bundles/day)	Height (cm)	Lean body weight (kg)	Hemoglobin (g/100 ml)	Serum albumin (g/100 ml)
40 – 50	19	115.1	160.7	42.46	16.2	4.06
50 – 60	24	130.6	165.3	48.79	15.6	4.07
≥60	3	145.7	167.3	56.23	16.3	4.08

[a] Analysis of the production data by the analysis of variance technique has shown that there was a significant difference ($p < 0.01$) for production between body weight groups shown in the table.

was a remarkable consistency in the work output of each individual worker, when measured over a period of 3 months, and the average production could be taken as representing the individual's work capacity. There were significant differences between body weight groups and their work output (see Table 3). Biochemical parameters were similar in all three groups.

Correlations between work output and different anthropometric parameters are given in Table 3. Work output was found to be related to weight as well as to height. However, when the influence of weight was partialed out, work output was not significantly related to height. Correlation between weight and work output was higher when the influence of height was partialed out. Work output was also highly correlated with lean body weight computed from the anthropometric data. Work output by these workers was not correlated with socioeconomic factors, such as family size, age, length of service, or family income.

The rates of work before and after lunch during an 8-hr shift by the workers with different body weights are given in Table 4. It can be seen that not only the total daily output, but the rate of production was also higher in higher body weight groups. It can also be seen that in each weight group, the rate of production after the meal was higher than before the meal.

The data presented here demonstrate that there are considerable individual differences in work output among the workers. If malnutrition is one of the underlying causes for the observed individual differences, the differences could be caused either by the current nutritional status or by the previous nutritional status of the workers. As judged by serum albumin, hemoglobin, and clinical status, the workers were not suffering from any nutritional deficiencies. These workers received regular medical care and were routinely receiving vitamin and mineral supplements. In addition, they received a substantial meal during the

Table 3. Correlation between productivity, weight, height, and lean body weight ($N = 46$)

Characteristic	Production 1	Weight 2	Height 3	Lean body weight
1 Production		0.72^b	0.43^a	0.74^b
2 Weight			0.51^b	0.98^b
3 Height				0.59^b

Partial correlations:
$r < 13.4 = 0.0279$ $r < 13.2 = 0.1095$ NS
$r < 14.3 = 0.6599^b$ $r < 12.3 = 0.6477^b$
$r < 14.2 = 0.2133$ NS $r < 12.4 = 0.1115$ NS
$^a p < 0.01$ (not statistically significant—NS)
$^b p < 0.001$

Table 4.   Rate of work per hr during the first shift[a] ($N = 46$)

Body weight (kg)	Bundles/hr		Mean production (bundles)/day
	Before meal	After meal	
40 – 50	15.3	17.0	119.6
50 – 60	16.7	19.6	132.4
≥60	17.8	20.8	141.1

[a] The first shift consisted of a 4-day period.

working shift that provided 1,240 kcals and 25 g protein. It is thus clear that immediately before and during the study their nutritional experience was satisfactory. Differences in work output could not therefore be attributed to differences in their current nutritional status.

There was, however, a significant correlation between body weight or lean body weight, on the one hand, and work output, on the other. The work outputs by workers with lower body weight were significantly less than those observed in workers with higher body weights. It has been shown by Viteri (1971) and Spurr, Barac, and Maksud (1974) that maximal work capacity is directly related to body weight or lean body weight. Spurr, Barac, and Maksud (1974) have also shown that maximal work capacity in poorly nourished individuals with low body weight could be improved after nutritional rehabilitation. Whether submaximal work capacity corresponding to real life work situations is also related to body weight has not so far been clearly demonstrated. In a recent study among sugar cane cutters by Spurr, Barac, and Maksud, work output measured in terms of amount of sugar cane cut was related to the nutritional status of the worker as judged by their body weight and height. The work performed by the sugar cane cutters can be considered as heavy physical activity. The present study provides evidence that even submaximal work capacity corresponding to moderate activity is related to body weight, and work output decreases with a decrease in body weight. The higher work output by the higher body weight group was observed to be caused mainly by a higher rate of work. It was also observed that the rate of work increased after a meal in all the groups, indicating the beneficial effects on productivity of providing a good meal during working hours. A similar observation was made by Spurr and co-workers among sugar cane cutters in whom work output was found to be higher after lunch than before lunch.

It is generally considered that low body weights and heights have a nutritional basis. There is evidence to suggest that as a result of inadequate food intake in early childhood, body weights and heights may not reach the full genetic potential (Vijayaraghavan, Singh, and Swaminathan 1971; Young, 1971; Hanumantha Rao and Satyanarayana,

1976). One may perhaps assume that these workers with lower body weight studied here suffered from inadequate food intake in early childhood.

The present data, therefore, suggest that a nutritional situation that leads to low adult body weight may be associated with reduced adult work output. The practical significance of this observation in any population with chronic malnutrition in early childhood is obvious. It must, however, be emphasized that only one type of work situation was investigated in the present study. Before the conclusions of this preliminary study can be accepted as being universally true, it is necessary to extend these studies to other work situations. This is currently being undertaken.

REFERENCES

Bhavani, B. 1966. Nutrition and efficiency in agricultural labourers. Indian J. Med. Res. 54: 971.

Damon, A., and Goldman, R. F. 1964. Predicting fat from body measurements: Densitometric validation of ten anthropometric equations. Hum. Biol. 36: 32.

Food and Agricultural Organization of the United Nations (FAO). 1962. Relation between diet and working capacity. In Nutrition and Working Efficiency. F.F.H.C. p. 13. Basic study no. 5, Rome.

Hanumantha Rao, D., and Satyanarayana, K. 1976. Nutritional status of people of different socio-economic groups in a rural area with special reference to pre-school children. Econ. Food Nutr. 4: 237.

Keller, W. D., and Kraut, H. A. 1962. Work and Nutrition. In G. H. Bourne (ed.), World Review of Nutrition and Dietetics, p. 65. Pitman Medical Publishing Company, London.

Satyanarayana, K., Hanumantha Rao, D., Vasudeva Rao, D., and Swaminathan, M. C. 1972. Nutrition and working efficiency in coal miners. Indian J. Med. Res. 60: 1800.

Siri, W. E. 1956. Body composition from fluid spaces and density. Report 19, Donnor Lab. of Med. Physics, University of California Berkeley, Ca.

Spurr, G. B., Barac, M. N., and Maksud, M. G. 1974. In Clinical and subclinical Malnutrition: Their influence on the capacity to do work. Annual Progress Report to Agency for International Development. Project No. AID/CSD 2943, 29 and 48.

Vijayaraghavan, K., Singh, D., and Swaminathan, M. C. 1971. Heights and weights of well-nourished Indian school children. Indian J. Med. Res. 59: 648.

Viteri, F. E. 1971. Considerations on the effect of nutrition on the body composition and physical working capacity of young Guatemalan adults. In N. S. Scrimshaw and A. M. Altschul (eds.), Amino Acid Fortification of Protein Foods, p. 350. MIT Press, Cambridge.

Young, H. B. 1971. Measurement of possible effects of improved nutrition on growth and performance in Tunisian Children. In N. S. Altschul and A. M. Altschul (eds.), Amino Acid Fortification of Protein Foods, p. 395. MIT Press, Cambridge.

Nutrition and Performance of Different Occupational Groups

K. Ošancová

Sportsmen have been interested for at least 2,000 years in the effect of nutrition on sports performance (Åstrand, 1970). It is safe to say that although these efforts are very old, an unequivocal answer to the question is still lacking. Workers have received less attention because their employers have traditionally shown little interest in the effect nutrition might have on working performance, and even less interest in workers' health status. Perhaps empirical experience taught them what Lehmann (1961) confirmed by scientific methods, i.e., that the relationship between performance and nutrition holds only in times of food shortage, and not when food is plentiful.

In investigations of the nutritional status of the population, attention was focused primarily on food intake, and data on the energy output were obtained from the literature. Recommended nutrient allowances were established for different occupational groups based on a combination of food consumption data from epidemiological surveys and data from the literature pertaining to the energy and nutrient requirements of different groups. There are, of course, certain difficulties associated with these procedures. When formulating recommended allowances it is recognized that those for children and adolescents must take into account requirements of growth and development of the organism. Furthermore, there must be special allowances for pregnant and lactating women and for old people.

As far as the adult population is concerned, views on the most suitable classification for purposes of recommended allowances are not so uniform. Some allowances take into account body weight, others age, and some specify in detail the work load, which is used as the main criterion of classification. In previous recommended allowances for adults (Hejda, Ošancová, and Mašek, 1971), the basis of classification was the work load, regardless of age within the range of 18–65 years.

Another factor that renders the elaboration of allowances difficult was pointed out by Ketz and Maune (1968), who maintained that there is a certain leveling off as far as the energy output in different occupations is concerned. In their opinion, the decrease in energy output that occurred in many occupations is compensated for by a greater energy output during leisure hours. According to this author's findings, leveling off of energy output in different occupations has actually taken place, but unfortunately it cannot be confirmed that the decrease is compensated for by more active recreation, sports activities, etc.

Durnin (1966, 1970, 1975) also referred to a decline in the energy expenditure in different occupations. He observed that in occupations classified as heavy work, the strenuous work actually takes up only short periods of time. He also pointed out that the energy expenditure in the same occupation differs greatly for different subjects, and therefore, the classification by occupation involves various inaccuracies. The same nominal occupation does not necessarily imply the same energy output. More detailed analysis revealed that the total energy output correlated closely with the output during working hours, but not with the output during the nonworking period.

The classification into groups in the last revision of recommended allowances and their calculation is based on the results of epidemiological surveys and on data from the literature. Working loads in the allowances are divided within both sexes into several categories— sedentary and light work (1); moderately active (2); and very active (3). For men there is an additional category: exceptionally active (4). In all categories subjects have been divided by age into a younger group, ages 19–34 years, followed by groups from 35–59 years in men and from 35–54 years in women. The classification of the older groups takes into account retirement age (Hejda et al., 1976).

For illustration, a few examples of the classification of different occupations are given: 1—student, tailor, photographer, clerk, housewife with a household of two; 2—actor, barber, chimney sweeper, farmer in agricultural cooperative, bus driver, hospital physician with night duties, waitress, housewife looking after a household of three or four; 3—stoker, engine driver on steam locomotive, ballet dancer, housewife looking after a household of five or more members; 4—miner, lumberjack, etc.

These classifications are only approximate and it is not possible to estimate accurately the energy output during work nor the output during nonworking hours.

Figure 1 illustrates schematically the trend of energy consumption in three groups of workers as recorded in large representative population groups during epidemiological surveys in 1970–1972.

I **sedentary or light work**
II **moderately active**
III **very active**

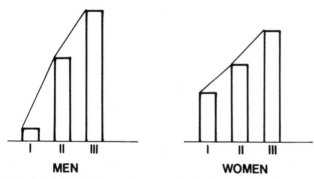

Figure 1. Trend of energy consumption in three occupational groups.

The trend of energy intake and animal protein and fat consumption in the same population classified by age are shown in Figure 2. A similar trend was recorded for the minerals investigated, i.e., calcium and iron, and to a lesser extent for the vitamins.

From both Figures 1 and 2, it is apparent that occupation, as well as age, exerts a marked influence on energy consumption, and it is therefore correct to take into account both criteria when preparing recommended allowances.

The example of heavy workers studied in one survey shall be used to demonstrate the results obtained by the author's method of investigation (Ošancová and Hejda, 1974).

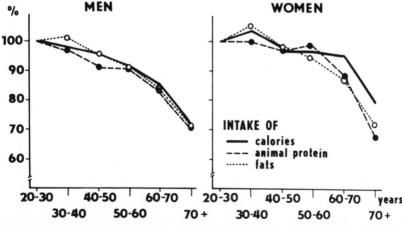

Figure 2. Energy intake and animal protein and fat consumption in population classified by age.

The group was investigated from 1970 to 1972 with the objective of obtaining data to specify the recommended allowances for heavy workers. This was of importance because views on the work load of some occupations are controversial. Although some authors maintain that as a result of technical progress and automation strenuous physical work is an exception, others overestimate the actual energy expenditure of some occupations.

A group of 159 subjects in occupations considered to require strenuous work were studied. The group included workers from: a) engineering industries (furnacemen, foundrymen, forgemen operating power hammers, metal plate cutters, etc.), b) brickmaking plants, c) transport industry (workers who load and unload railroad cars), d) mining industry, and e) meat packing houses.

At the start of the experiment, subjects were administered a comprehensive examination (Hejda and Ošancová 1967, 1969, 1970). It consisted of a standard clinical and somatometric examination, and an assessment of food consumption by a modified inventory method, which involves the biochemical indicators of the nutritional status. In addition, the hemoglobin and ascorbic blood levels (Bessey, Lowry, and Brock, 1947) and serum cholesterol (Grafnetter et al., 1967) were measured.

The clinical findings revealed the heavy workers to have a higher incidence of subclinical signs of malnutrition in otherwise healthy subjects. As far as pathological conditions were concerned, spondylogenic changes, hypertension, and gastroduodenal ulcers predominated.

Among somatometric findings, the relatively high incidence of overweight persons and obesity deserve mention. Severe obesity, i.e., more than 125% of the desirable weight, was observed in 21.4% of the subjects. The incidence was lowest among workers in the brickmaking plant (5%) and highest among butchers from the packing house (35%) as

Table 1.   Percentage of incidence of overweight and obesity in heavy workers

	Above 105% desirable weight	Above 115% desirable weight	Above 125% desirable weight
1. Heavy engineering	68.5	35.2	17.6
2. Workers from brick plant	52.6	21.0	5.2
3. Transport workers	61.1	33.3	25.0
4. Miners	50.0	18.7	12.5
5. Butchers	70.3	56.8	35.2
1 − 5 ($\bar{X}$)	63.6	36.5	21.4

shown in Table 1. This incidence is high even when compared with formerly investigated groups of miners, foundry workers, etc.

Overweight and obesity in different occupational groups of heavy workers rise with the average age of the group, although the average energy intake declines with advancing age.

The energy consumption of the investigated groups varied between 3,700 kcal and 5,082 kcal. The lowest mean consumption was recorded in butchers and the highest in workers from the brickmaking plant, where intakes as high as 7,000 kcal were found. The consumption, with the exception of vegetable proteins, carbohydrate, and vitamin C, was above the recommended level.

Among biochemical findings, the serum cholesterol level as compared with the representative population group from Bohemia and Moravia was significantly higher in miners and significantly lower in the other occupational groups.

The hemoglobin level in the groups was relatively low—23.9% of the heavy workers had hemoglobin levels below 14 g/100 ml, while the corresponding ratio in a representative sample of the Czech male population ages 18 to 64 years was 11%.

A synthesis of the clinical, somatometric, food consumption, and biochemical findings reveals that many heavy workers overestimate their energy expenditure and their caloric intake is excessive, resulting in overweight and obesity. However, it must be realized that mean figures mask the considerable interindividual differences in food consumption.

On the other hand, as may be concluded from the high incidence of signs of malnutrition, the investigation revealed that demands on the composition of the diet for subjects working in an adverse environment are higher than for subjects with a similar energy expenditure working under more favorable conditions. Of special importance are nutrient losses by perspiration, as pointed out by Heinrich et al. (1966).

Among the occupational groups of heavy workers, the working conditions of the furnace chargers and dischargers in the brickmaking plants were the most demanding, because very strenuous work is combined with an adverse working environment.

Epidemiological surveys revealed that although it is not possible to use laborious methods for assessment of the energy expenditure in field studies, the rough classification system used in this experiment provides very useful information. Estimates of the energy expenditure in field studies must take into account not only the nature of the work but the age of the worker. Furthermore, loss of nutrients by perspiration must be considered when workers are under adverse climatic or microclimatic conditions.

REFERENCES

Åstrand, P. O. 1970. Nutrition and physical fitness. Proc. VIIIth Int. Nutr. Congr., Prague, 1969, pp. 44–50. Publ. Excerpta Medica, Amsterdam.

Bessey, O. A., Lowry, O. H., and Brock, M. J. 1947. The quantitative determination of ascorbic acid in small amounts of white blood cells and platelets. J. Biol. Chem. 168: 197–205.

Durnin, J. V. G. A. 1966. Age, physical activity and energy expenditure. Proc. Nutr. Soc. 25: 107–119.

Durnin, J. V. G. A. 1970. Energy expenditure in relation to age, sex, body weight and physical activity. Proc. VIIIth. Int. Nutr. Congr. Prague, 1969, pp. 321–323. Excerpta Medica, Amsterdam.

Durnin, J. V. G. A. 1975. Unresolved problems in establishing international standards for energy requirements. Proc. IXth Int. Congr. Nutr., Mexico, 1972, Vol. 1, pp. 35–42. Karger, Basel.

Grafnetter, D., Fodor, J., Teplý, V., and Žáček, K. 1967. The effect of storage and levels of cholesterol in serum as measured by a simple direct method. Clin. Chim. Acta. 16: 33–37.

Heinrich, H. C., Gabbe, E. E., Meineke, B., and Whang, D. H. 1966. Biologische Halbwertzeit und Umsatzrate des Eisens im Gesamtkörper des Menschen. (Biological half-life and turnover of iron in the human body.) Klin. Wochenschr. 44: 904–906.

Hejda, S., and Ošancová, K. 1967, 1969, 1970. Vývoj výživové situace u našeho obyvatelstva. (Development of the nutritional status of our population.) Final report. Institute of Human Nutrition, Prague.

Hejda, S., Ošancová, K., Kajaba, I., Bučko, A., Grunt, J., and Malík, A. 1976. Nové výživové doporučené dávky pro ČSSR. (New recommended nutrient allowances for the ČSSR.) Výživa Lidu. 31: 17–20.

Hejda, S., Ošancová, K., and Mašek, J. 1971. Nový návrh doporučených výživových dávek. (New recommended nutrient allowances.) Čas. Lék. Česk. 110: 1153–1156.

Ketz, H. A., and Maune, R. 1968. Der Energieverbrauch von Industriearbeitern verschiedener Berufsgruppen. (Energy consumption of industrial workers with different occupations.) Ernährungsforschung 13: 1–6.

Lehmann, G. 1961. Lehrbuch der gesamten Arbeitsmedizin. 1. Arbeitsphysiologie. Urban und Schwarzenberg, Berlin.

Ošancová, K., and Hejda, S. 1974. Health and nutritional status of heavy workers. Rev. Czech. Med. 20: 76–84.

Occupational Activities and Nutritional Status in West Germany

W. Wirths

The energy expenditure of the occupational activities in all industrial countries has decreased, particularly during the last 20 years of industrialization. In West Germany, most occupational persons have a better nutritional status than those in earlier times. A high percentage of the workers are obese. Many of them are engaged in sedentary work (an estimated 25% or more).

Two kinds of methods are used for assessing the development of the project: indirect evaluation with calculation of the occupational activities, and direct assessment of the energy requirements and the energy and nutrient intake.

INDIRECT METHOD OF ASSESSING
ENERGY EXPENDITURE AND NUTRIENT INTAKE

Indirect evaluation of the classification of occupations (Durnin and Passmore, 1967; Durnin et al., 1973) and international comparison of the corresponding categories is provided by the "International Standard Classification of Occupations 1968" (ISCO) of the International Labour Organization (ILO) (1969). For assessing these values, the energy and nutrient requirements of workers with different physical occupations and from different age groups, and the unemployed have been studied in many places with the Max Planck respirometer (Müller and Franz, 1952; Wirths, 1974). An attempt is first made by the indirect method to establish the mean nutrient and energy intake based on the average food consumption of the entire population. Then types of work and the whole population are categorized by age and occupation, and the energy and nutrient requirements with intake levels are calculated. The results are given in Table 1.

Table 1.   Consumer groups of the population in West Germany (1974)

Age group		N (in thousands)	Work group	N (in thousands)
Infants under 1 year		690	Light work	29,850
Children	1–3 years	2,440	Sedentary work	9,808
	4–6 years	2,980	Heavy work	2,686
	7–10 years	4,100	Very heavy work	298
	11–14 years	3,780	Pregnant women	650
Adolescents	15–20 years	4,220	Lactating women	170
Total population: 61,672,000				

DIRECT METHODS OF ASSESSING ENERGY EXPENDITURES, NUTRIENT REQUIREMENTS, AND NUTRITIONAL ANTHROPOMETRY

For the determination of the energy expenditure in respiration studies by work, the Max Planck respirometer was utilized. It is an instrument used in the field that consists of a small dry gas meter, weighing 2.5–3 kg, which is either carried on the back, like a haversack, or on the chest. The subject performs his usual work, and breathes through an expiratory valve. The expired air passes through the meter. The meter contains a device by which a small fraction of the expired air, about 0.3 to 0.6%, is diverted into a small rubber bag. This sample is subsequently analyzed.

Pulse rate measurements were taken in order to determine the rate of heartbeat occurring in professional activities. These were initially done in several population groups for the assessment of the circulatory system in static work. The method of heart rate alone is not used. The use of heart rate to predict energy expenditure has been shown to involve errors that may be as high as 10 to more than 30%, depending on the subject, the type of activity, the adaptation of training, and the body weight.

The assessment of total energy expenditure of workers not only depends on energy expenditure during working time but also on that during leisure time. Nonoccupational activities can be of substantial importance, considering the great number of working persons concerned, the proportion of occupational energy expenditure, and total work calories. It was found especially in a number of employees, particularly in situations of light and moderate work, that these people do much work during their leisure time at various seasons of the year: for example, house or garden work, house mechanics and repairs, and sports. The worker benefits from performing these tasks.

SECONDARY CONSIDERATIONS
IN ASSESSING ENERGY EXPENDITURES

In view of the decreasing total energy expenditure of the population, different factors are important. First, the increasing mechanization and the high degree of automatization in work places during recent years is evident. Less physical work needs to be done because of progressing mechanization. In several work places, during a period of 8 to 10 years, there was sometimes found a decrease of 0.5–1.5 working kcal per min. During a whole shift this amounts to about 500 kcal. Sometimes the decrease found in 8 hr was only 100 kcal. Workers in the latter category were more overweight in the second period of the examination.

Therefore, in West Germany a similar problem to that in other industrialized countries exists: a tendency for a large percentage of the people to favor light work, mainly sedentary activities with small amounts of energy expenditure. Moreover, although most individuals work five days per week, they are working fewer work hours and fewer work days because of a greater number of holidays. There are typically more jobs for females. The age limit is younger and the percentage of older people in the working population is greater.

The dietary patterns, or course of the nutritional status, of the population during the last few decades are virtually the same as those existing in other countries comparable from our industrial standpoint. Durnin and Passmore (1967), Consolazio (1972), Wretlind (1975), and den Hartog (1975) have all reported the same trend for the working people. In the Federal Republic of Germany there has been a decrease in the consumption of grain products, principally rye flour and bread, and potatoes. At the same time there has been an increase in obesity, both the visible and invisible (hidden) fat. Another change in the food intake during the last few years is an increase in the consumption of products rich in animal protein. Most of this group of foods has a higher fat content. Furthermore, the consumption of sugar and sweets has increased, as has that of vegetables and fruit. There also has been a considerable increase in minor contributions to the diet of various luxury commodities—particularly cream, ice cream, chocolate, chocolate and sugar mixed products, soft drinks, potato products, peanuts, and other such snack foods, all rich sources of calories. Last, but not least, the consumption of alcoholic beverages has increased to an average of about 300 kcal per person per day. The total number of all German foodstuffs is about 5,000 items. There are, for instance, more than 200 kinds of bread.

There has also been a remarkable increase in the number of items of food consumed per week. In the period from 1950–60, the number per

Table 2.   Energy and nutrient supply in West Germany (per capita and day)

Nutrient		1946/47	1972/73	1972/73 (% change from 1946/47)
Protein from	(g)	72	83	115
animal	(g)	26	55	212
Fat	(g)	44	140	318
Carbohydrate	(g)	368	350	95
Energy	(kcal)	2,085	2,980	143
	(MJ)	8.7	12.5	

capita per week was, on the average, 26 items. Since 1970, the average number of food items consumed in more than 15,000 case histories ranged from 8 to 108 items. Elderly people and people from lower socioeconomic groups had a more restricted diet.

The development of the nutritive and energy level for the average of the entire population of the Federal Republic of Germany since 1946 is shown in Table 2. The notable aspects are the noticeable increase in energy content, animal protein, and fat. During this same period, the protein content has remained nearly constant and the carbohydrate intake has decreased. In percentages, the energy content without calories of alcoholic beverages is protein, 11.4; fat, 44.0; and carbohydrate, 44.6. The 44% fat calories are divided into 21% saturated fatty acids, 18% monounsaturated, and 5% polyunsaturated.

The 300 calories of alcoholic beverages contain 10% protein, 40% fat, 41% carbohydrate, and 9% alcohol. There is an increase in all minerals and vitamins, and on the average all nutrients are balanced. In food purchases, one may consider a 20% waste in vitamins A, B_1, and B_2, and a 50% waste in vitamin C.

Not all individuals have a balanced nutrient status. Therefore, direct methods were used to study the nutritional status of special groups of the population. First, the energy expenditure and nutritional anthropometry for most occupations varied widely. All work for men and women was divided into groups according to the energy expenditures, as shown in Table 3. After this classification, about 70% of all workers have energy expenditures that classify them as light workers; about 23% are moderate or sedentary workers. The rest are heavy and very heavy workers (Table 4).

One of the most important groups from the standpoint of ergonomics is the office workers, mostly those in administrative services, with sedentary work and minimal body movement. Occupational energy expenditures are of little importance because of the sub-

Table 3.   Work group and sex

Work group	N (in thousands)	Male (%)	Female (%)
Light work	29,850	39	61
Sedentary work	5,858	60	40
Heavy work	2,686	86	14
Very heavy work	298	100	

jects' sedentary occupations. Consequently, in many of the subjects, energy expenditure as a result of movement is higher in nonworking periods. Sometimes nonoccupational energy expenditures are found to exhibit surprising differences. Some volunteers increased their total energy expenditure by about 600 kcal/day because of their nonoccupational activities. With increasing energy intake, total amounts of protein and animal protein increased, but, in most cases, the energy intake decreased at the same time.

The energy input is for most persons higher than required—not only when the energy balance is positive, but also when it is equalized in static obesity. One-third of the volunteers were overweight. Three methods were utilized for the evaluation of the degree of overweight. For males a simple formula is recommended: height $\times$ 400 = weight in g; for *female*: height (cm) $\times$ 350 = weight in gram ($\pm 5\%$).

The energy output of the people engaged in sedentary work shows decreased and reduced dynamic muscle work. In most work studies, the net occupational energy output in sedentary workers was less then 20 kcal/hr. On the average there was a great discrepancy between the energy expenditure and energy value of food intake. However, most of the subjects' meals, as revealed by precise weighing methods, showed

Table 4.   Working groups of employed persons, including housewives

Working group	1882 (%)	1925 (%)	1950 (%)	1975 (%)
Light worker	21	24	58	70
Sedentary worker	39	39	21	23
Heavy worker	26	25	16	6.3
Very heavy worker	14	12	5	0.7
Employed person (Millions)	16.9	32.0	32.2	39.8
Population total (Millions)	45.7	63.2	50.0	61.7

a high rate of waste in the foods purchased, which amounted to 15-25%.

It can be concluded and estimated that the whole population of West Germany has a rate of waste of about 10-12% for all food. Some experiments were performed and it was found that the waste generally was small for alcoholic beverages, eggs, and citrus fruits, but high in the cases of fats and oils and other products with high hidden fat content. Vegetables also showed a large waste. No one knows the exact amount of the different foodstuffs lost on the way to the consumer and the waste by the consumer.

In view of the nutritional status of the entire population, it can be said that there is sufficient money available for adequate nutrition for all groups. Elderly people, persons being rehabilitated after accidents, and the people on social welfare, as well as the unemployed are able to have adequate nutrition. The number of unemployed at the end of June, 1975 was one million. Of these, 57% were male and 43% female. Most people have a poor knowledge of nutrition. Others know about adequate nutrition, but the taste and the flavor of the food are the elementary reasons for consumption.

Many people in affluent nations require far less energy for everyday life, particularly in cases when less physical work is needed. However, the actual energy intake is seldom appropriate to the individual's real need, and the surplus has an adverse effect on his health. Overeating and insufficient muscular work not only encourage growth of body fat deposits, but may also contribute to the development of diseases because of complications arising from obesity. Most of these complications are serious diseases such as diabetes, abnormalities of the vascular system, diseases of the gall bladder, varicose veins, and difficulties with the joints as a result of continous overloading of the bones and joints.

In this situation, the appetite-regulation mechanism in man is significant. Lehmann's (1951) metabolic reduction in higher animals indicated it is commendable that the energy intake is less than two times that of the basal metabolic rate. Animals, apparently, do not grow fat when living in the wilds. Most animals have a work load in proportion to their energy uptake and their basic metabolic rate. Mayer et al. (1954) demonstrated with rats that when activity was increased involuntarily by walking on a treadmill, the spontaneous energy intake (food being available ad libitum) was directly correlated with the work load. Their body weight then remained constant. If their activity was restricted, the animals ate relatively more and became obese. Contrary to this, they ate less and lost weight when exercising. In man, all energy intake above the basal metabolic requirement must be within a certain range of "normal" activity. The level, twice the metabolic rate, is not reached in our active population. The relation in more than 70% of our exercising persons is less than 1:0.5 between basal metabolic rate and other energy expenditure, in moderate workers 1:0.8, in heavy workers 1:1.2, and in very heavy workers 1:1.5.

Another result in these experiments is the high protein intake when food is available ad libitum. It was found in steel workers, blast furnace workers, and lumber workers, all with a total energy expenditure of 4,000 kcal per person per day or more, that they have an adequate nitrogen balance in a formula diet with 1 g protein per kg body weight. It was difficult to give only 75–90 g protein per day in such an energy rich diet. However, in these same groups, it was found that the protein reserves decreased in nearly all the exercising people. It was measurable in the mid-arm muscle circumferences. Their upper arm circumferences decreased, but the skinfolds of the biceps and triceps did not. Therefore, the muscle mass decreased. When they had a formula diet of 1.5–1.8 g protein or more per kg body weight, protein content was constant or increased, and the percentage in upper arm muscle circumference was constant or increased. The same was found to be true of a small group of sportsmen (rowers) during the period before the last Olympic Games (Wirths, 1972).

The development of the cardiac and vascular diseases through arteriosclerotic processes bears some relation to the composition of the blood. Not only diet and physical activity but hereditary factors, high blood pressure, and stress as a result of psychic factors are highly conducive to the incidence of cardiovascular complaints.

Greater physical activity and a limitation of the intake of foods rich in fat, mainly saturated fatty acids, available carbohydrates, and alcohol, are recommended. This leaves more room in the diet for protective foodstuffs, protein, polyunsaturated fatty acids, vitamins, and minerals. It involves less risk of partial nutrition, particularly for people who have an intake of less than 2,000 kcal energy per day. Furthermore, one should also avoid excessive consumption of foods rich in cholesterol. This author disagrees heartily with Durnin et al. (1973) that it is possible for a group of healthy subjects with similar attributes and activities to have nutrient and energy intakes that vary as much as twofold without making any difference in their body weight. A decrease in the quickness and the effective quantity of motion during work and in leisure time were first noted. Furthermore, the body weights are a decisive influence.

Steady state is reached when the energy expenditure is constant— i.e., performing the same kind of work over a long period. Above that level, nearly all people will be slow or very slow in their body movements. If a body weighing 65 kg has a steady state of 4.2 kcal/min, then one weighing 102 kg has a steady state of only 2.3 kcal/min (55% less).

Last, but not least, using a Douglas bag technique, it was found that there is a decrease of 10−25% in the adaptation of the basic metabolic rate, even after small amounts of movement in different groups of workers (mainly sedentary workers). This was true of not only elderly persons but also of middle-aged and younger people.

SUMMARY

Over the last 20 years, the energy expenditure of more than two-thirds of the population in West Germany has decreased. Less physical work needs to be done because of progressing mechanization. The tendency of a large percentage of the people is to favor light, mostly sedentary, work. Moreover, there is presently more leisure time. Most workers have a five-day work week that is continually decreasing. There are also more jobs for females.

The dietary patterns and food habits are in a longitudinal evolution. On the average, the intake in unavailable carbohydrate is decreasing, and the readily available carbohydrate level is increasing. The intake in fat, animal protein, minerals, vitamins, and energy is also increasing.

It is recommended that in addition to greater physical activity, a limitation be imposed on the intake of foods rich in fat—mainly saturated fatty acids, available carbohydrates, and alcohol. This involves less risk of partial nutrition, particularly for people who have an intake of less than 2,000 kcal/day. Furthermore, one should avoid excessive consumption of foods rich in cholesterol.

REFERENCES

Consolazio, C. F. 1972. Nutritional status and work capacity relationships. Aliment. Trav. 1: 227−245. Masson et Cie., Paris.

den Hartog, C. 1975. Food and nutrition in the Netherlands. World Rev. Nutr. Diet. 22: 1−39. Karger, Basel.

Durnin, J. V. G. A., Edholm, O. G., Miller, D. S., and Waterlow, J. C. 1973. How much food does man require? Nature 242: 418.

Durnin, J. V. A., and Passmore, R. 1967. Energy, Work and Leisure. Heinemann, London.

International Labour Organization. 1969. International Standard Classification of Occupations—ISCO, ILO Genf.

Lehmann, G. 1951. Das Gesetz der Stoffwechsel reduktion in der höheren Tierwelt. (The law of metabolism reduction in higher animal species.) Z. Naturforsch. 6b: 216−219.

Mayer, J., Marshall, N. B., Vitale, J. J., Christensen, J. H., Mashayekhi, M. B., and Stare, F. J. 1954. Exercise, food intake and body weight in normal rats and genetically obese adult mice. Am. J. Physiol. 177: 544.

Müller, E. A., and Franz, H. 1952. Energieverbrauchsmessungen bei beruflicher Arbeit mit einer verbesserten Respirations-Gasuhr. (Measurement of energy consumption during professional work with an improved gasometer.) Arbeitsphysiologie 14: 499–504.

Statistisches Bundesamt 1968. Internationale Standardklassifikation der Berufe. (Federal Statistical Office, International Standard Classifications of Professions.) Deutsche Ausgabe. (German edition.) Verlag W. Kohlhammer, Stuttgart, und Mainze, 1971.

Statistisches Bundesamt. 1970. Klassifizierung der Berufe, systematisches und alphabetisches Verzeichnis der Berufsbenennungen. (Federal Statistical Offices, Classification of Professions, Systematic and Alphabetical List of Professional Titles.) Verlag W. Kohlhammer, Stuttgart und Mainz.

Statistisches Jahrbuch über Ernährung, Landwirtschaft und Forsten. (Statistical Yearbook of Nutrition, Agriculture and Forestry.) Parey, Hamburg, und Berlin, jährlich.

Wirths, W. 1972. Energie- und nährstoffzufuhr von hochleistungssportlern. (Energy and nutrient supply of high performance sportsmen.) Sport. Sportmed. 23: 253–256.

Wirths, W. 1974. Evaluation of energy expenditure and nutritional status in dietary surveys. Bibl. Nutr. Diet. 20: 77–91.

Wretlind, A. 1975. Future trends in parenteral nutrition. Bibl. Nutr. Diet. 21: 177–195.

Nutrition, Exercise, and Health

Effects of Diet or Diet and Exercise in Weight Reducing Regimens

J. Šonka

The wartime exhaustion caused by a reduced food intake, mental stress, and hard work was soon compensated for in Czechoslovakia after the last war by an outbreak of obesity. A weight reducing regimen with a relatively rich caloric intake (1,800 kcal a day) and very moderate physical activity, installed in all hospitals and baths, turned out to be ineffective, especially in cases of long-term obesity, already adapted to a reduced food intake.

METHODS

This postwar situation led to the proposition 18 years ago of introducing a new regimen with a rather strict diet (Šonka and Přibylová-Čarková, 1977) and heavy physical activity. The diet (900 to 1,000 kcal a day) had the following composition: 70 to 75 g proteins, 45 g fats, and 65 to 70 g carbohydrates (mainly vegetables and fruits). Noncaloric beverages were not restricted. The following scheme of physical activity, directed by qualified instructors, was followed: 2 hr of gymnastics and ball handling drills in the morning, and in the afternoon some competitive games and water sports were on the program (2 hr). After dinner, dance or rhythmic exercises were offered. These combined summer regimens (C) of 13 days were organized in sports centers or in baths equipped with all the necessary facilities (Šonka and Žbirková, 1963). The winter regimen of 7 days took place in the mountains, with skiing as the main physical activity. Evenings were occupied by rhythmic exercises and dances. Anorectics and diuretics were not administered, and sauna and other heat procedures leading to dehydration were not recommended.

This regimen was open to all obese subjects recommended by their district physician, who was requested to complete a form containing limited but vital information about the proposed participant, as well as a list of contraindications pertaining to cardiovascular and locomotor diseases. The age limits were 17 to 45 years. The admitted patients were not compelled to follow the regimen strictly.

RESULTS

Metabolic Effects

For the estimation of energy expenditure, the telemetric recording of the pulse rate was used (Rouš et al., 1973). The calculated mean energy deficit of 3,500 kcal was designed to produce a loss of about 390 g fat daily. However, the summer regimen (C) led to a weight loss of 4 to 4.5 kg, while a loss of 2 to 3 kg was obtained in a regimen with an identical diet and a small, spontaneous physical activity (Regimen D). This difference between the expected and actual weight loss in Regimen C may have been attributable to sex (90% of the patients were women), height, and overweight of the patients. Tall and considerably overweight men lost as much as 10 kg in summer. The lowest weight loss (1 to 2 kg) was observed in small women with a body weight approximately equal to the upper limit of normal values. If the weight loss was considered in relation to overweight, a more important weight loss was obtained by overly obese subjects. After a rapid weight loss during the first few days, the decrease of body weight slowed down and an increase of 1 or even 2 kg sometimes appeared at the end of the first week, but afterwards the daily weight losses were again quite regular (Doberský, Doleček, and Šonka, 1967). This was principally the result of a significantly positive nitrogen balance (Figure 1), not present in Regimen D (Slabochová et al., 1962). Similar effects of intense physical activity were also seen in men, but to obtain a positive nitrogen balance, an intake of at least 1,400 kcal was needed (Štěpánek and Křižek, 1971). The retention of nitrogen was caused by an enhanced proteosynthesis, especially in the liver and muscles. Because up to 6 g of water may be bound to 1 g of protein, even a small change in body protein influences body weight. The loss of sodium and water as a result of reduced efficiency of aldosterone is another mechanism involved in the weight loss during the first days of such a regimen.

The skinfold measures (Figure 2) indicated a decrease of subcutaneous fat proportional to the thickness of the skinfold (the maximal decrease of fat was found on the abdominal wall), although the maximal work was requested from the largest groups of muscles (thigh). There existed no special exercises designed to decrease the volume of

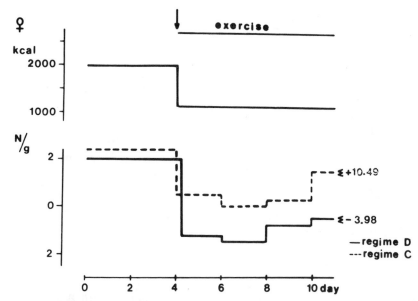

Figure 1. Nitrogen balance in obese women. Regimen C featured diet and exercise, Regimen D featured only diet.

the fat pads in specific body locations, because the lipomobilization depends on hormones brought to the lipocytes by blood vessels. In many body parts no neural or humoral communication exists that

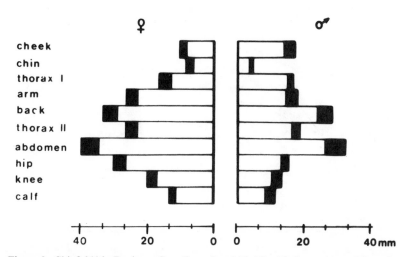

Figure 2. Skinfolds in Regimen C on Days 0 and 12. The black portions of the column represent the decrease in the skinfold measurements caused by the treatment.

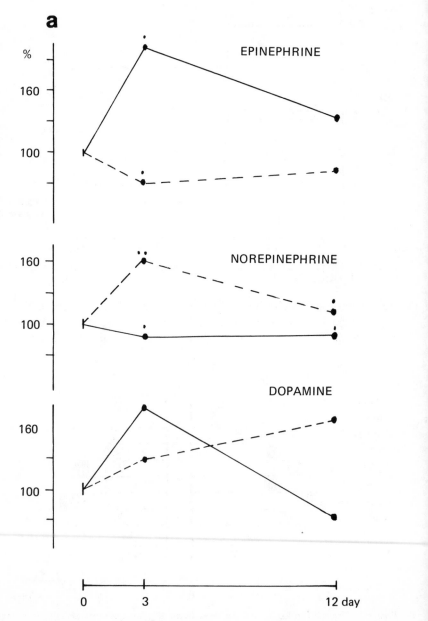

Figure 3. Epinephrine, norepinephrine, and dopamine excretion in Regimens C and D (a). Vanilylmandelic acid and creatinine excretion in Regimens C and D (b).———Regimen D,----Regimen C. · $p < 0.05$, ·· $p < 0.01$.

transmits information directly from the working muscle to the superimposed fatty tissue. A similar effect of Regimen C on fat redistribution may be evaluated in exercising obese subjects from simple measurements of body circumferences (Šonka et al., 1965). Therefore, the role of some proteosynthetic, lipolytic, and liposynthetic factors was studied in both regimens.

Regimen C led especially on Day 3 to an enhanced excretion of epinephrine, whereas no change was observed in Regimen D. On the other hand, norepinephrine excretion was increased in Regimen D, but no effect was observed in Regimen C. Both of the regimens had no significant effect on dopamine excretion (Šonka et al., 1974). The excretion of 4-Hydroxy-3-methoxymandelic acid (vanillylmandelic

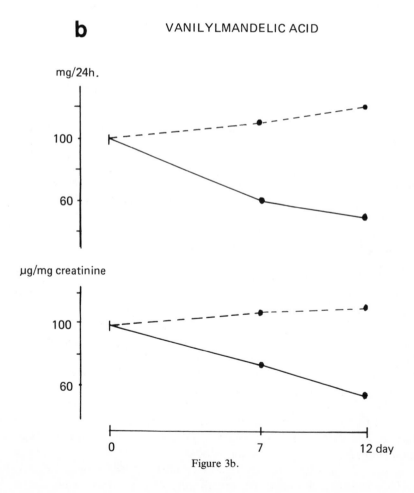

Figure 3b.

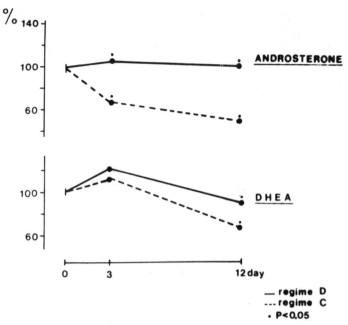

Figure 4. Androsterone and dehydroepiandrosterone (DHEA) excretion in Regimens C and D.

acid) was decreased in Regimen D, and the difference between the Regimens C and D was significant from Day 3 until Day 12 (Šonka and Petrášek, 1963). The different effects of diet (D) and of the combined regimen (C) on catecholamine excretion did not confirm the hypothesis of a simple additive effect of two lipomobilizing stimuli in Regimen C, e.g., food restriction and physical activity (Figure 3).

The basal morning values of somatotropin (STH) in the group following Regimen D led to a twofold increase in Days 3 and 12, but in Regimen C the increase was minor. STH is generally estimated immediately after a stimulus (e.g., physical activity, fasting), but in these experiments blood was obtained after a night's rest. This time interval between the stimulus (exercise) and the secretory bouts of STH may be the main reasons why the results in a group of 11 patients were opposite to the expected trend (Sonka et al., 1974a).

The proteoanabolic effect of muscular activity may be attributable to such factors as the plasma level of two adrenal androgens, androsterone, and dehydroepiandrosterone (DHEA). Androsterone in Regimen D progressively decreased to a point of 50% of the initial value. In Regimen C the initial serum level was maintained through the test. DHEA followed a similar pattern (Figure 4). The decreasing serum content of adrenal androgens in the case of energy deficit enhances the catabolism of muscle proteins—on the other hand, muscular activity accompanied by an even larger energy deficit is good protection against protein catabolism. It should be mentioned that DHEA is an inhibitor of glucose-6-phosphate dehydrogenase. Hence, a decreased serum level of DHEA may lead to an enhanced lipid synthesis (Šonka et al., 1972). This is another factor that should be taken into consideration when discussing the role of physical activity as an integral part of weight reducing programs.

Plasma cortisol levels were assayed in both regimens and no significant changes were found on Days 0, 3, and 12.

The effect of Regimen C was also tested on glycemia and insulinemia 30 min after an oral load of 100 g glucose. The rise of glycemia had a similar trend before and after the 12-day regimen; the post-treatment mean values on Day 0 and Day 12 were only 4 mg/100 ml lower. The rise of insulinemia (IRI) was somewhat lower at the end of the regimen (a rise from 12.2 to 31.5 μU) in comparison to the values obtained before starting the regimen (11.5 to 38.9 μU/ml). The recorded differences in both glycemia and insulinemia were not significant.

The effects of Regimens C and D on the activity of the pentose phosphate cycle (PC) were studied in erythrocytes because no other more convenient tissue for metabolic studies was available. The PC values in normal, nonobese women were in the range of 7 to 8% of the total amount of utilized glucose, but the initial value of PC in obese women was elevated to 12%. A decrease occurred beginning with the first day in both regimens, but the rate of decrease was greater in Regimen C. The reduction of PC was of short duration, however, and on Day 14 the values of PC returned nearly to the initial levels. The elevated PC values in erythrocytes of obese women may be considered to be a metabolic stimulus to lipogenesis in tissues not involved in triglyceride synthesis. On the other hand, the decrease of PC is a deterrant to liposynthesis because of a reduced supply of extramitochondrial NADPH (Šonka and Slabochová, 1960).

Physical Fitness

Physical fitness was also studied in Regimen C. The vital capacity, the hand grip strength, and the abdominal muscle strength were evaluated. On starting the regimen, the vital capacity in the men was 98% of ideal values, and reached a value of 105% after 12 days of the regimen. A similar rise from 90 to 97% was obtained in obese women. The hand dynamometer presented a significant improvement; however, no increase of strength of abdominal muscles was observed. The test chosen for abdominal muscles was too easy for most of the patients. Further tests consisted of a run of 50 and 200 m, a bimanual underhand shot put, and a standing hop, step, and jump. There was a tendency toward improvement in women in the 200 m race and in putting the shot, and a significant improvement was obtained in the triple jump (increase of 16.0 ± 6.5 cm). These events were not involved in the training program during the course of the experimental treatment. The favorable effect of Regimen C was also documented by a combined step test as described by Kříž et al. (1972) and Žbirková, Kříž, and Šonka (1973). The patients were required to step on two steps, one 10 and one 20 cm high, in a definite rhythm for a fixed time. The sum of the pulse rates resulting from stepping up and down from the two banks decreased from 320.6 ± 40.4 to 303.5 ± 42.4 after treatment. These results were obtained from 400 obese women.

The patients were also followed by a psychologist who confirmed personal observations that Regimen C enhanced the motivation, reduced the depressive moods, and supported the patient's decision not to abandon this new mode of daily living.

SUMMARY AND CONCLUSION

The effects of 12 days of diet (Regimen D) or of diet combined with physical activity (Regimen C) were studied in obese subjects. In Regimen C, an important weight loss was obtained in spite of the presence of proteosynthesis, because of a positive nitrogen balance and support by adrenal androgens. In Regimen D, the nitrogen balance had a tendency to negative values and the plasma androgens decreased. The protection of lean body mass in Regimen C was also documented by skinfold measurements.

Plasma hydroxycorticoids and serum somatotropin were not affected in either regimen under the conditions of this experiment. In Regimen D an increase of epinephrine excretion was present; in Regimen C an enhanced excretion of norepinephrine and of vanillylmandelic acid was recorded. There was no change in dopamine excretion in either regimen. A tendency toward a decrease of insulinemia and glycemia was observed in Regimen C if pre- and post-treatment values were compared, but the results were not significant. A greater decrease of the participation of the pentose phosphate cycle in erythrocyte glucose metabolism was observed in Regimen C, but a return to nearly initial values occurred in both regimens on Day 12.

Physical fitness was studied only in Regimen C, which led to an increase in vital capacity and of hand grip strength and to a decrease of pulse rate in a combined step test. A tendency to amelioration occurred in the 200 m run and in bimanual underhand shot put; a significant increase was obtained in a standing hop, step, and jump.

The presented results, including psychological benefit, suggest that physical activity is an indispensable complement of diet in the treatment of obesity, with exclusion of severe cardiopulmonary or joint complications.

REFERENCES

Doberský, J., Doleček, R., and Šonka, J. 1967. Léčení otylosti, p. 153. (Treatment of obesity.) SZdN Praha.

Kříž, V., Šonka, J., Žbirková, A., and Taichmanová, Z. 1972. Tělesná výkonnost otylých žen. Výsledky dvoustupňové funkční zkoušky oběhové. (Physical fitness of obese women. Results of a combined step test.) Vnitř. Lék. 18: 644–651.

Rouš, J., Kočnár, K., Kříž, V., and Žbirková, A. 1973. Použití telemetrie k hodnocení intensity pohybového režimu otylých. (The use of telemetry for the determination of energy expenditure in exercising obese subjects.) Prac. Lékař. 25: 300–303.

Slabochová, Z., Placer, Z., Mašek, J., Rath, R. and Šonka, J. 1962. Metabolismus u obésních. (Metabolism in obese subjects.) Čs. Gastroenterol. 16: 230–236.

Šonka, J., Gregorová, I., Tomsová, Z., Pavlová, A., Žbirková, A., and Josífko, M. 1972. Plasma androsterone, dehydroepiandrosterone and 11-hydroxy-corticoids in obesity. Effects of diet and physical activity. Steroid Lipid. Res. 3: 65–74.

Šonka, J., Kopecká, J., Pavlová, A., and Žbirková, A. 1974a. Catecholamines excretion and plasma growth hormone in obese women. Effects of diet and physical activity. Symposium über Lipidstoffwechselerkrankungen, Dresden, Teil II, pp. 521–525.

Šonka, J., Kopecká, J., Pavlová, A., Žbirková, A., and Staš, J. 1974b. Effects of diet and exercise on catecholamine excretion. Horm. Metab. Res. 6: 532.

Šonka, J., Křížek, V., Štěpánek, P., Kučerová, M., and Žbirková, A. 1965. Svalová činnost a redukční režim. (Exercise and weight reduction.) Vnitř. Lék. 11: 245–261.

Šonka, J., and Petrášek, J. 1963. Vliv redukčních režimů na vylučování 3-metoxy-4-hydroxymandlové kyseliny (vanilmandlové). (Effects of weight reducing regime on the excretion of vanilmandelic acid.) Čs. Gastroenterol. 17: 430–434.

Šonka, J., and Přibylová-Čárková, M. 1977. Dieta Při Otylosti. (Reducing Diet.) 6th ed., p. 70. Avicenum, Prague.

Šonka, J., and Slabochová, Z. 1960. Der Glycidmetabolismus bei Obesen bei Reduktionsdiät und der Einfluss des Dexfenmetrazins. (Glucose metabolism of the obese treated with diet and the influence of dexfenmetrazine.) Endokrinologie 40: 75–84.

Šonka, J., and Žbirková, A. 1963. Pohybem a dietou proti otylosti. (The role of exercise and diet in a slimming regime.) SZdN, Praha.

Štěpánek, P., and Křížek, V. 1971. Vliv cvičení na bílkoviny těla při redukci váhy. (Effects of exercise on body protein in weight reduction.) Rehabilitácia 4: 131–138.

Žbirková, A., Kříž, V., and Šonka, J. 1973. Změny tělesné výkonnosti otylých žen při 14ti denních letních rekreačních pobytech pro otylé. (Effect of a weight reducing regimen on physical fitness of obese women.) Teorie Praxe Těl. Výchovy 21: 3–7.

Effects of Voluntarily Restricted Diets on Physical Fitness in Sedentary Work Conditions

M. Apfelbaum, A. Reinberg, F. Duret

In a society of food abundance, a great part of the population feels obese. Consequently, there follow periodic, relatively severe, restricted diets. However, the notion of strength associated with food intake is so powerful that the restricted diets are often accompanied by absences from work in order to "rest." This chapter attempts to examine the objective basis for such a behavior by providing information only on moderately obese subjects whose work calls for limited physical efforts. Thus, the conclusions cannot be extrapolated, either to subjects who are chronically undernourished, or to work conditions involving great effort.

SUBJECTS, MATERIALS, AND METHOD

A group of nine apparently healthy but obese women (18 to 25 years of age) volunteered for this study during a 3-week hospitalization period. These subjects were overweight by 10 to 30%, according to the Metropolitan Life Insurance Company Standards of 1959. A set of testing procedures was used to estimate circadian changes in physiological and psychophysiological variables before and during a so-called 220 cal protein diet (Apfelbaum et al., 1967; Apfelbaum, Bostsarron, and Brigant, 1969; Apfelbaum et al., 1970; Apfelbaum et al., 1971; Apfelbaum, 1973). In order to compensate for the nitrogen lost, 55 g of protein in the form of calcium caseinate were administered daily (220 cal). The diet also included 1.5 liters of desalted water, a polyvitamin mixture, and 2.0 g of potassium bitartrate. The mean weight loss after 3 weeks was 7.60 kg.

Isocaloric "meals" were served at fixed hours (0800, 1300, and 2030). The subjects were socially synchronized with a diurnal moderate activity, from about 0700 to about 2300, and a nocturnal rest. The chronobiologic effects of such a diet in similar experimental conditions and subjects have been reported. Circadian changes in oxygen consumption and respiratory quotient, plasma HGH, insulin, glucagon, and cortisol, among other physiological variables, have been demonstrated (Apfelbaum et al., 1971, 1972; Reinberg, Apfelbaum, and Assan, 1973).

Measurements were performed over a 24-hr period once a week every 6 hr, at fixed times (0600, noon, 1800, and midnight) before (i.e., nonrestricted spontaneous food intake) and during the 3-week, 220 cal protein diet.

On specially prepared sheets, the subject had three series of meter shaped horizontal rectangles equal in size with a scale from 0 to 5. Each series was used for the *self-rating of hunger, mood, and physical vigor*. The subject was told that any rectangle might be likened to, for instance, the speedometer of a car. She was asked to indicate her estimation of the amount by a pencil stroke; the farther to the right the pencil mark appeared, the higher was the rated estimate of the variable. With these self-rated estimates repeated at fixed clock hours over a 24-hr period, circadian changes in hunger, mood, and physical vigor could be documented, including the 24-hr mean. These self-rating tests, although quite simple, proved to be very reproducible with only small noise in rhythm detection (p 0.005) (Simpson et al., 1971; Reinberg et al., 1973).

Self-measurements concerning the following tests were performed, and the results were recorded at each of the test times:

1. *Grip strength* of the right hand was measured using a Colin Gentile dynamometer. The mean of five measurements was recorded.

2. The *fatigue test* also involved the dynamometer to evaluate the subject's fatigability. This was measured by the decrease in grip strength during a standardized repeated effort. The subject was instructed to take 20 consecutive readings of his grip strength and to record each of them. The values obtained in each group of five were averaged. The first series of five measurements provided an observation of the reference mean for grip strength. The last series revealed the level of fatigue when compared with the individual reference mean.

3. *Eye-hand Coordination* was determined by the use of a stop watch to measure the time taken to transfer 30 metal bearings from the palm of one hand to a small tin box, inserting them into a vertical tube with a diameter just sufficient to admit them when inserted "end on."

4. *Tempo* was assessed by using the stop watch face down. The subject measured the time necessary to count from 1 to 120 (evaluation of a 2 min span of time).
5. *Rectal temperature* was recorded from a calibrated medical thermometer (scale in 0.1°C).

The time series obtained were first analyzed using conventional statistical methods in order to check whether the curve resulting from the time-plotted data followed, at least roughly, a sine function. This was the case, so the cosinor method was used for both rhythm detection and characterization. The latter included the acrophase, $\emptyset$, the peak of the best fitting sine function approximating all data; $\emptyset$, the midnight reference, in keeping with the subjects' synchronization; the amplitude, A, one-half of the 24-hr total within individual variability; and the mesor, M, the 24-hr rhythm adjusted mean which in this case was equal to the arithmetical mean, since measurements were performed at equal intervals and fixed times. When the considered rhythm was determined ($p \leq .05$), $\emptyset$ and A were given with their respective 95% confidence interval; M was given $\pm$ 1 SE.

RESULTS

The data are summarized in Table 1 and in Figures 1 ($\emptyset$'s) and 2 (mesors).

The results related to the hunger self-rating were expressed in arbitrary units. The acrophase in the sensation of hunger occurred shortly before 0600. The average feeling of hunger over 24 hr (mesor) was not modified by 15 days of protein diet. However, it dropped significantly during the third week, confirming the impression gained from nonquantitative clinical studies that very restrictive diets produce no increase in the sensation of hunger when compared with the spontaneous ad libitum diet. In contrast, moderately restrictive diets (1,200 cal, for example) are known to induce a persistent feeling of hunger. A remarkable feature here was the marked drop in the feeling of hunger when the protein diet was prolonged. Both mood and physical vigor self-rating showed a transient fall in M, which occurred during the second week of the diet.

Muscular Strength and Fatigability

Muscular strength was not altered by the protein diet, at least insofar as grip was concerned. This finding was confirmed by fatigue measure-

Table 1. Circadian rhythms in physiologic variables of healthy but obese young women before and during caloric restriction (220 cal/24 hr protein exclusively)

Physiologic variables[a]	Before sd and after 2 or 3 weeks of cr[b]	Rhythm detection (p)	Rhythm-adjusted level (M ± 1 SE)	Amplitude (hr/100 MJ)[c]	φ Acrophase (hr, min)[d]
Hunger, SR (arbitrary)	sd	<0.010	476 ± 51	16 (±9)	0558 (0002 – 1154)
	2 weeks cr	<0.010	451 ± 49	14 (±9)	0559 (0003 – 1158)
	3 weeks cr	<0.005	264 ± 27	10 (±5)	0558 (0500 – 0654)
Mood, SR (arbitrary)	sd	<0.005	169 ± 14	14 (±10)	1918 (1855 – 1941)
	2 weeks cr	<0.005	142 ± 8	11 (±8)	0557 (2358 – 1146)
	3 weeks cr	<0.005	160 ± 13	12 (±9)	0554 (2356 – 1144)
Physical vigor, SR (arbitrary)	sd	<0.005	152 ± 12	13 (±7)	1912 (1830 – 1954)
	2 weeks cr	>0.005	120 ± 11	11 (±7)	0600 (0042 – 1118)
	3 weeks cr	<0.005	142 ± 14	13 (±8)	0548 (2353 – 1143)
Grip strength,[e] SM	sd	<0.025	92 ± 1.2	6 (±5)	1159 (0647 – 1711)
	2 weeks cr	>0.5	90.7 ± 2.8		1102
	3 weeks cr	<0.005	91.6 ± 3.1	6.7 (±3)	1107 (0704 – 1509)
Fatigue test, SM[f]	sd	<0.025	84 ± 1.8	6 (±5)	1405 (0827 – 1942)
	2 weeks cr	<0.5	82.3 ± 2.7		1348
	3 weeks cr	<0.5	82.4 ± 2.1	6.5 (±5.5)	1336 (0806 – 1907)
Eye-hand coordination,[g] SM	sd	<0.005	88 ± 3	7 (4 to 11)	0253 (0055 – 0451)
	2 weeks cr	<0.005	86 ± 4	6 (3 to 9)	0248 (0218 – 0407)
	3 weeks cr	<0.005	86 ± 4	5 (2 to 9)	0135 (2232 – 0443)
Tempo, SM (count from 1 to 120 sec)	sd	<0.05	142 ± 7	5 (1 to 9)	1356 (0929 – 1824)
	2 weeks cr	<0.005	139 ± 5	8 (2 to 14)	1527 (1227 – 1827)
	3 weeks cr	<0.025	137 ± 4	7 (1 to 13)	1711 (1341 – 2042)
Rectal temperature (C), SM	sd	0.005	36.99 ± 0.88	0.8 (±0.3)	1624 (1400 – 1848)
	2 weeks cr	0.005	36.81 ± 0.19	0.8 (±0.3)	1548 (1258 – 1838)
	3 weeks cr	0.005	36.90 ± 0.09	0.8 (±0.3)	1556 (1224 – 1929)

[a] Self-rating (SR), self-measurement (SM).

[b] Spontaneous diet (sd), caloric restriction (cr).

[c] 95% confidence interval.

[d] Acrophase reference: midnight.

[e] First set of five. Grip strength is expressed for each individual as percent of the value measured at the acrophase when the subject is in spontaneous diet. At each fixed clock hr grip strength was measured and recorded 20 times within 40 sec. Data thus obtained were averaged in four consecutive series of five. Presented results are restricted to the first and the fourth set of measurements (muscular fatigue test).

[f] Grip strength, fourth set of five measurements.

[g] Eye-hand coordination was the time taken to transfer 30 metal bearings from the palm of one hand to a small tin box by inserting them into a tube with a diameter just sufficient to admit them when inserted end on. The acrophase corresponded to the longer span of time (sec) to perform the test. Obviously, the best skill is located 12 hr before or after the acrophase.

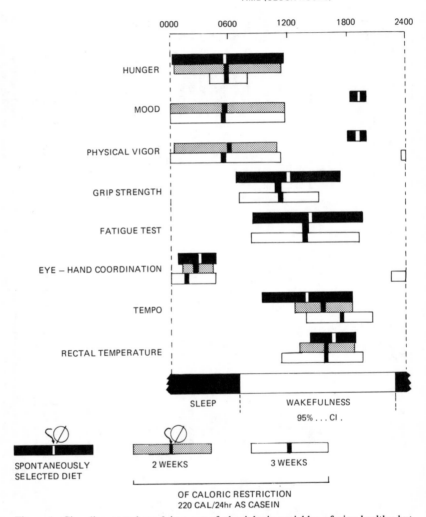

Figure 1. Circadian acrophase Ø in a set of physiologic variables of nine healthy but obese young women before and during 3 weeks of the 220 cal protein diet.

A statistically Ø shift of ~ 12 hr occurred only in both the circadian rhythms of hunger and mood self-rating, when comparing Ø estimates before and during the experimental diet. Ø's of other investigated variables show neither any diet-induced shift nor consistent difference with respective Ø locations resulting from similar studies performed in healthy human adults.

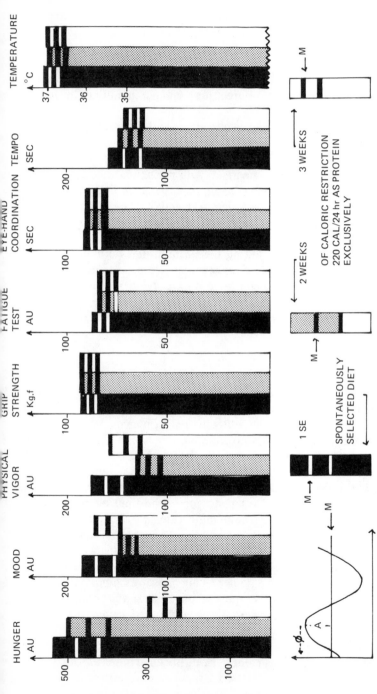

Figure 2. Circadian rhythm adjusted mean M in a set of physiologic variables of nine healthy but obese young women before and during 3 weeks of the 220 cal protein diet.

A statistically significant diet-induced fall (~ 55% during the third week) occurred in the hunger self-rating, M. It can be related to a change in the fuel used by the brain (ketone bodies instead of carbohydrates).

A transient fall (occurring only during the second week of the diet) was observed also in both mood and physical vigor self-rating, Mesors (M). The mesors of the other variables did not show any statistically significant change.

As a whole, these results favor the conclusion that the 220 cal protein diet is not likely to disturb the subject's fitness for non-strenuous work.

ments, which likewise were not affected by the diet. There is no statistically significant variation in the mesor of fatigue.

Eye-Hand Coordination

The time required to perform the eye-hand coordination test was not longer, nor was the hour of poorest performance modified, during the protein diet.

Both tempo and temperature circadian rhythms were not altered by the diet.

Thus, apart from tempo and oral temperature, circadian rhythms reported here permitted a comparison with previous studies, the results of which can be divided into two categories: the quantification of subjective feelings clearly related to cerebral activity, i.e., self-ratings of hunger, mood, and physical vigor; and neuromuscular performances.

The two sets of findings reveal notable differences. "Subjective" performances were altered during the protein diet, with an important decrease in the circadian M of hunger, and a transient decrease in the circadian M of physical vigor and mood. Neuromuscular performances, on the contrary, underwent no alteration. However, it should be noted that the tests called for only a moderate effort from the subject.

DISCUSSION

In another experiment, using the same type of subjects (moderately obese, healthy women) and the same diet (protein diet), the effects of meal timing were studied. The following performances, using the same tests as in the present study, were compared between spontaneous and protein diet: when subjects consumed their total intake for breakfast, when they consumed all of their intake for dinner, and when they consumed it in four isocaloric meals. Again, no change was found in the mean value of the performances nor in the time of the subjects' maximal performances. The results may seem surprising in view of the fact that such a diet induces a huge change in fuel circulation. The muscles shift from an occasional use of fatty acids to a systematic use of this fuel. The brain shifts from the exclusive use of glucose to a predominant use of ketone bodies. One must remember that these results concern only limited muscle use; when the subjects were studied during bicycling exercises, there was a considerable drop in their normal power.

The diet studied was exclusively protein and was compared to a mixed diet at a spontaneous caloric level. Because there was no drop in performances, the results can be extrapolated to any restricted diet between the habitual intake and 220 cal/day. However, they cannot be extrapolated to shifts in meal timing with no caloric restriction. Preliminary results obtained with young healthy subjects eating their usual amount of food but with a different meal pattern suggested that their mean performances and the time of maximal performance were modified.

CONCLUSION

The 220 cal protein diet decreases hunger, does not alter mood and physical vigor, and results in no change in any of the tests for fitness for nonstrenuous work, despite the modification of energetic nutrients used by the organism. Such a diet (and probably all less severe restricted diets) is compatible with continued sedentary work. Obviously, this conclusion must be limited to activities for which the battery of tests used gives pertinent information. It cannot be extended to activities such as hard manual labor or competition.

REFERENCES

Apfelbaum, M. 1973. Influence of level of energy intake in man: Effects of a spontaneous intake experimental starvation and experimental overeating obesity. Proceedings of the meeting on obesity. US Printing Office, Washington, D.C.

Apfelbaum, M., Bostsarron, J., Brigant, L., and Dupin, H. 1967. La composition du poids perdu au cours de la diète hydrique; Effets de la supplémentation protidique. (Composition of weight loss during a water diet; Effects of protein supplements.) Gastroentérologie 108: 121–134.

Apfelbaum, M., Bostsarron, J., and Brigant, L. 1969. La diminution de la consommation "basale" d'oxygène sous l'effet d'une restriction calorique chez des sujets en bilan d'azote équilibré. (Decrease in basal metabolism due to restriction of caloric intake in subjects having a nitrogen balance.) Rev. Française Etude Clin. Biol. 14: 361–372.

Apfelbaum, M., Bostsarron, J., and Lacatis, D. 1971. Effect of caloric restriction and excessive caloric intake on energy expenditure. Am. J. Clin. Nutr. 24: 1404–1409.

Apfelbaum, M., Boudon, P., Lacatis, D., and Nillus, P. 1970. Effets métaboliques de la diéte protéique chez 41 sujets obèses. (Metabolic effects of protein diets in 41 obese subjects.) Presse Méd. 78: 1917–1920.

Apfelbaum, M., Reinberg, A., Lacatis, E., Abulker, Ch., Bostsarron, J., and Riou, F. 1971. Rythme circadien de la consommation d'oxygène et du quotient respiratoire de femmes adultes en alimentation spontanée et aprés restriction calorique. (Circadian rhythms of oxygen consumption and respiratory quotient of adult females on spontaneous diets and after caloric restriction.) Rev. Europ. Etude Clin. Biol. 16: 135–143.

Apfelbaum, M., Reinberg, A., Assan, R., and Lacatis, D. 1972. Metabolic and hormonal circadian rhythms before and during a 200 cal/24 h protein diet. Israël J. Med. Sci. 8: 867–873.

Cahill, G. F., Herrera, M. G., Morgan, A. P., Soeldner, J. S., Steinke, J.,

Levy, P. L., Reichard, G. F., and Kipnis, D. M. 1966. Hormone fuel interrelation during fasting. J. Clin. Invest. 45: 1751.

Felig, P., Marliss, E., and Cahill, G. F. 1973. Metabolic pathways in starvation. "Régulation de l'équilibre énergétique." Paris 1: 83–94.

Goetz, F., Bishop, J., Halberg, F., Sothern, P. B., Brunning, R., Senske, B., Greenberg, B., Minors, D., Stoney, P., Smith, L. D., Rosen, G. D., Cressey, D., Haus, E. and Apfelbaum, M. Timing of single daily meal influences relations among human circadian rhythms in urinary cyclic AMP and jemic glucagon, insulin and iron. Experientia 32: 1081–1084.

Halberg, F. 1965. Some aspects of biologic data analysis: Longitudinal and transverse profiles of rhythms. Circadain Clocks Proc. J.: 13–22.

Reinberg, A. 1974. Chronobiology and nutrition. Chronobiologia 1: 22–27.

Reinberg, A., Apfelbaum, M., Assan, R. 1973. Chronophysiologic effects of a restricted diet (220 cal/24h as casein) in young healthy but obese women. Int. J. Chronobiol. 1: 391–404.

Simpson, H. W., Kelsey, C., Gatti, R. A., Good, R., Halberg, F., Bohlen, J. G., Sothern, R. B., Delea, C. S., Haus, E., and Bartter, F. C. 1971. Autorhythmometry in myasthenia gravis; Detection of chronopathology and assessment of condition by rhythm adjusted level of grip strength. J. Interdisc. Cycle Res. 2: 397.

Physical Activity, Nutrition, and Cardiovascular Diseases

R. Masironi

PHYSICAL ACTIVITY AS A CARDIOVASCULAR HEALTH FACTOR

Cardiovascular diseases are the major cause of death in industrialized countries, not only in elderly subjects but also in younger, highly productive age groups. Mortality rates from ischemic heart disease are apparently associated with living standards and have increased during the last few decades. Proportionally higher increases are noted in relatively younger age groups, e.g., 35–44 years (WHO, 1969).

Life table analyses show that during the last decades there has been a declining trend in life expectancy for men (about 8 years), which seems to be caused to a great extent by ischemic heart disease. It is commonly held that the increase in cardiovascular mortality is attributable at least in part to a pattern of increasingly sedentary life. The economically less privileged populations that lead a physically more active life are almost free from myocardial infarction. However, this pattern is changing as technological progress resulting in sedentary and other harmful life habits also reaches the developing countries.

To what extent is it anecdotal, and how much scientific truth lies in the belief that physical activity is good for the health, particularly for the health of the heart?

The crucial problem to be studied is: does physical activity have a preventive influence on the development of ischemic heart disease? If this is the case, what are the mechanisms involved and which types and amounts of exercise are required?

Epidemiological Evidence
from Industrialized Population Groups

Evidence of allegedly beneficial health effects of physical activity comes mostly from epidemiology, which, however, cannot yield any proof of causality.

Since Morris et al. (1953) published their authoritative paper on the role played by sedentary living habits on the incidence of myocardial infarction, many investigators have attempted to discover

257

if physical inactivity was really a risk factor for coronary heart disease. Froelicher and Oberman (1972) made a critical survey of 35 published reports, but were unable to find a satisfactory degree of consistency among the investigations.

Fletcher and Cantwell (1974) took a more optimistic view, but were still unable to demonstrate conclusively that exercise or a physically active life lowers the incidence of coronary heart disease.

Table 1 shows that generally beneficial trends of physical activity on cardiovascular health are reported by many authors, but several other studies did not reveal such trends.

The discrepancies in the results are to a great extent the results of lack of standardization in all these independent, uncoordinated studies. Moreover, whatever results were found in a given population, they cannot be generalized and extrapolated to other population groups without adjusting for differences in life habits, diet, smoking, psychosocial background, and other pertinent factors.

The relationship between physical activity at work and cardiovascular disease was studied recently by a highly standardized method in well-defined population groups (Kagan et al., 1977). In this post-mortem study, internationally coordinated by WHO, subjects who engaged in strenuous physical work showed less aortic and coronary atherosclerosis, less coronary stenosis and thrombosis, and less frequent myocardial infarction and myocardial scars than sedentary subjects. Although causality cannot be ascertained in this study, Kagan et al., infer the existence of "an association of atherosclerotic and myocardial lesions with sedentary work, and an inverse association with strenuous work."

Rissanen (1976) also found that men in occupations demanding regular physical activity and heavy exercise had less extensive coronary atherosclerosis at autopsy than men in sedentary occupations, and fewer electrocardiographic abnormalities compatible with myocardial ischemia were detected in a group of middle-aged male executives who reported exercising vigorously (Epstein et al., 1976).

In conclusion, men in physically active jobs generally seem to have a lower incidence of coronary heart disease in middle age than men in sedentary occupations, and, if they do have a coronary event, the disease is usually not as severe.

Epidemiological Evidence from Nonindustrialized Population Groups

Many studies on nonindustrialized physically active population groups consistently report low prevalence of atherosclerosis and of myocardial infarction (see Fejfar and Masironi, 1970, for references). The classic study of Mann et al. (1965) on the Masai pointed to the role of large amounts of exercise, mostly walking, to explain the fact that the Masai men did not show clinical signs of cardiovascular disease of the atherosclerotic type. An example of particular interest is the comparative study of the health of two groups of Cook Island Maoris. One group lives under town conditions (Rarotonga) with a marked amount of social pressure and changes typical of a "westernized" type of life, and the other lives in an isolated atoll (Pukapuka). The Pukapukans' daily calorie intake is 85% of that of the Rarotongans, and they have a higher daily physical activity level. Concurrently they have less obesity, much less atherosclerosis, and almost no hypertension as compared with the Rarotongans, among whom these conditions are, instead, becoming highly prevalent (Prior et al., 1966).

The findings of these two, by now rather old, studies are confirmed by other, very recent investigations. For instance, the ECG abnormalities found in Canadian Eskimos are much fewer than those of the U.S. population, and are very seldom of ischemic type. Aortic calcification is also much less prevalent in Eskimos (Hildes et al., 1976). In rural populations of Eastern Siberia, the incidence of myocardial infarction is very low, and Sedov (1976) emphasizes the role played by "constant manual labour and nutrition no more than adequate to meet energy losses" in explaining the low morbidity from myocardial infarction in the rural populations of Eastern Siberia. Regular physical activity associated with a slightly low dietary intake (2,500 kcal/day, i.e., 10.4 MJ/day) of Peruvian Quechua Indians is thought to be responsible to a great extent for the absence of hypertension and for the low serum cholesterol values of these people (Watt et al., 1976a).

Evidence from Physical Rehabilitation of Postmyocardial Patients

An enormous amount of literature is available on physical rehabilitation of postmyocardial patients, and it would be outside the scope of the present chapter to even attempt to review it. Useful information is contained in Fletcher and Cantwell (1974).

The opinions are discordant, however. Sometimes it seems that physical rehabilitation is of no major preventive usefulness, as far as subsequent occurrence of another myocardial infarction and age of death are concerned. In other instances, clear-cut beneficial results have been obtained. Although there is really no hard evidence that physical rehabilitation lessens morbidity and mortality from coronary heart disease, physical rehabilitation is commonly thought to be of both physical and psychological benefit, because it eliminates the

Table 1. Epidemiology studies: Physical activity and coronary heart disease (CHD)

Type of study	Principal investigator	Occupations	Correlation of physical activity with lowered risk of CHD
England-Wales mortality	Morris	Different occupations	Yes
London transport	Morris	Drivers versus conductors	Yes
North Dakota	Zukel	Farmers versus others	Yes
American railroad	Taylor	Switchmen versus clerks	Yes
Italian railroad	Menotti	Switchmen versus clerks	Yes
South African railroad	Adelstein	Different occupations	No
Evans County, USA	McDonough	Laborers versus white collar	Yes
Health Insurance Plan of New York	Frank	Less active versus more active	Yes
Washington, D.C. postal employees	Kahn	Mail carriers versus clerks	Yes
Israeli kibbutzim	Brunner	Sedentary versus nonsedentary	Yes
West Virginia miners	Higgins	Miners versus nonminers	No
Peoples Gas Co., Chicago	Stamler	Blue collar versus white collar	Yes
California mortality	Breslow	Different occupations	Yes
Irish brothers	Brown	Work in USA versus work in Ireland	Yes

Harvard football	Pomeroy	Athletes versus nonathletes	Yes, in athletes who kept active after graduation
College oarsmen	Prout	Athletes versus nonathletes	No, but athletes lived longer
Danish athletes	Schnor	Athletes versus nonathletes	No, but athletes lived longer
Harvard athletes	Polednak	Athletes practicing 1 or 2 sports versus athletes practicing 3 sports or more	No; more CHD in athletes practicing three or more sports
San Francisco	Paffenbarger	Cargo workers versus clerks	Yes
Framingham	Kannel	Active versus sedentary	Yes
Gothenburg	Werko	Active versus sedentary	Yes, but only in nonsmokers
British Civil Servants	Morris	Active versus inactive	Yes, for leisure time activity
Seven countries	Keys	Active versus sedentary	No, at 5-year follow-up; yes, at 10-year follow-up[a]
East/West Finland	Karvonen	Sedentary versus lumberjacks	No, higher in lumberjacks
Western collaborative	Rosenman	More active versus less active in leisure	Yes
Western Electric, Chicago	Paul	Different occupations	No
Los Angeles civil servants	Chapman	Different occupations	No

Most of this data from Fletcher and Cantwell (1974), reproduced by permission from *Exercise and Coronary Heart Disease*, Charles C Thomas, Publisher.

feeling of invalidity and brings the cardiac patient back more quickly to his former job than is the case with patients who were not rehabilitated.

A comprehensive discussion of the benefits of physical rehabilitation following myocardial infarction is contained in a publication by the International Society of Cardiology (1973), based on the advice of a large number of experts from many countries. The conclusion is that the vast majority of patients who survive myocardial infarction can benefit significantly from relatively simple, safe, and inexpensive physical rehabilitation measures.

Mechanisms of Action

Although it is still debated whether or not exercise protects one from a coronary attack and/or prolongs life, physical activity certainly exerts a marked influence, both directly and indirectly, on the cardiocirculatory function.

Indirect influence may be exerted through the better life habits of health-minded, physically active people who perhaps smoke less, may tend to eat a more balanced diet, etc., while the direct physiological influence is hypothesized to occur through an increase in the mass, contractility, and vascularization of the cardiac muscle, supposedly induced by physical training.

Greater amounts of work can be performed by the trained heart, which utilizes oxygen more economically. Physical activity lowers the resting heart rate, and working performance is increased at a given heart rate. Certain physiological parameters that, when abnormal, are considered to be risk factors in the development of coronary heart disease, are seemingly "beneficially" influenced by exercise and fitness, e.g., serum triglyceride level, blood pressure, platelet activity, and obesity.

EFFECTS OF PHYSICAL ACTIVITY
ON CARDIOVASCULAR RISK FACTORS

Hypertension

Several studies have shown that systolic blood pressure decreased significantly after an exercise program, and physically more active men had lower systolic and diastolic blood pressure than sedentary men (Lange Anderson and Elvis, 1956; Pyörälä et al., 1967). In patients suffering from arterial hypertension, physical training programs have proved useful in normalizing blood pressure (Skinner et al., 1964; Gottheiner, 1968). These and other similar reports (e.g., Montoye et al., 1972; Morris et al., 1973) thus indicate a definite beneficial effect of physical activity on the regulation of the resting blood pressure.

Hyperlipidemia

Whether or not physical exercise lowers serum lipid levels is debatable, particularly as far as cholesterol is concerned. Several studies showed a decrease in serum cholesterol level following physical exercise programs, but there have also been many negative reports (see Fletcher and Cantwell, 1974, for reference). Other studies have shown little or no effect on blood cholesterol levels after exercise training unless body weight also was reduced through reduced dietary intake (Watt et al., 1976b). Montoye et al. (1976) found lowered levels of blood cholesterol and triglycerides in active subjects, but diet did not account for the differences. Hickey et al. (1975) found that physical activity during occupation did not bring about any differences in blood cholesterol and blood pressure. However, heavy activity during leisure time was associated with lower blood cholesterol and blood pressure.

Some of the contrasting results of serum cholesterol levels could be overcome by measuring the serum levels of high density lipoproteins (HDL), which are always elevated after an exercise program, unlike other lipoproteins. Because HDLs are the main carriers of cholesterol, increased HDL level suggests increased cholesterol turnover and removal (Miller and Miller, 1975).

Tendency to Thrombosis

Platelet activity and adhesiveness, which predispose to thrombus formation and possibly coronary occlusion when abnormally high, decrease during physical work while fibrinolytic activity increases, but there is no evidence that these apparently beneficial reactions last beyond the period of exercise to exert a long-lasting protective effect. On the other hand, short-term physical exercise results in increased platelet count, which would not be beneficial for subjects already at risk, particularly patients with a history of myocardial infarction (Sarajas, 1976). The effect of physical activity on the delicate balance between blood coagulation and fibrinolysis is not yet well understood.

Obesity

Of all the coronary risk factors of physiological and clinical nature, obesity is the one that is most closely interrelated with the two risk factors of behavioral nature that characterize modern, industrialized life habits: sedentariness and overnutrition. A combination of these two factors leads to an excess deposit of body fat.

Several investigators have shown that obesity is associated with a shortened life expectancy and with physical disorders, which are more frequent and more serious than in nonobese people. A recent autopsy study of atherosclerosis in five European towns, coordinated by the

World Health Organization (Kagan et al., 1977), showed that subjects with a great deal of subcutaneous fat had more atherosclerosis, especially of the coronary arteries, and a higher prevalence of coronary stenosis and myocardial lesions than those with little subcutaneous fat. The WHO Myocardial Infarction Community Registers (WHO, 1976) showed that at all ages the obese subjects had a statistically significant increase in the risk of dying, as compared with those of average build.

Obesity is not necessarily caused simply by overeating, but also by insufficient energy consumption. In the absence of exercise, however, eating less does not prevent the occurrence of obesity (Stefanik et al., 1959). The opposite is also true. Exercise alone will not decrease body fatness unless it is accompanied by dietary changes.

A study by Mayer et al. (1956) on sedentary and manual workers in India clearly demonstrated how increased physical activity in heavy physical work caused a proportional increase in food intake as compared to light work, but it did not bring about any increase in body

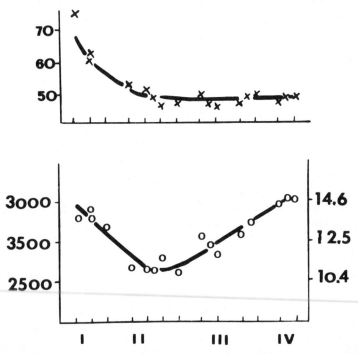

Figure 1. Body weight and caloric intake as functions of physical activity (J. Mayer et al., 1956). The upper graph ordinate is body weight (kg); the lower graph ordinates are caloric intake (kcal/24 hr) on the left, and caloric intake (MJ/24 hr) on the right. I indicates sedentary work; II, light work; III, medium work; IV, heavy work. Reproduced by permission.

weight. On the other hand, sedentary workers maintained the same caloric intake as the heavy workers, and their body weight was thus higher (Figure 1).

Discontinuation of physical training usually brings about an increase in body fat. This is particularly true for former athletes who were accustomed to eating abundant, protein-rich diets and continued to eat in approximately the same fashion in spite of having discontinued their physically active life.

Obesity is also a problem in child health, particularly in girls after puberty. Johnson et al. (1956) found a prevalence of 8.6% in American schoolboys and 12% in schoolgirls. Pařízková (1974) estimates that 10–15% of the children in the technologically advanced countries are obese. Obesity is primarily a problem in the industrialized, sedentary societies. When representative groups of children from highly industrialized and less industrialized countries are compared on the basis of skinfold thickness, it is evident that there is much more fatness among the children of the affluent societies (Figure 2). Pařízková (1974) found

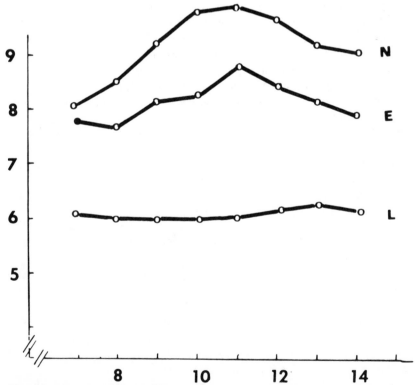

Figure 2. Obesity in boys of different countries (Lange Andersen et al., 1978). N = Norway, E = England, L = Libya. The vertical axis represents triceps skinfold thickness (mm), and the horizontal axis represents age (years).

widespread obesity among children of the upper socioeconomic classes in developing countries, also.

In conclusion, obesity should be considered as a borderline state of health and, consequently, prevention of obesity is an important part of public health programs.

NUTRITION

Nutrition, physical activity, and physical fitness are closely interrelated. Both undernutrition and overnutrition interfere with physical activity and fitness and lessen performance levels. For instance, Ethiopian boys, who are often undernourished (their daily caloric intake is only 70% of the FAO/WHO recommended values) have low functional development (Vo_2 max about 40 ml/min/kg versus 55 ml/min/kg of the better nourished Masai boys) (Mann et al., 1965; Lange Andersen, 1973).

Rural adolescents who subsist mainly on a diet excessively rich in carbohydrates and poor in animal proteins and fats have lower indices of physical status and of physical performance capacity than urban adolescents, whose diet is richer in proteins, fats, and calcium (Shirai, 1975). Small body size and weight under these dietary conditions of course, remain, through adult life, but eventually the rural adults, because of lifelong heavy physical work, develop a higher degree of physical fitness than the adult city dwellers. The latter eat a more balanced diet but are often obese from excessive calorie intake and are of inferior physical fitness because of limited physical activity. Obesity and heart diseases are common among them (Suzuki, 1975). The Tunisian boys from poor families studied by Pařízková (1974) had lower somatic development than the boys from wealthier families, but had higher functional capacities, better cardiovascular reactions during exercise, quicker postexercise recovery, less obesity, greater relative muscle strength, and better sports performance. This was caused most likely by a combination of adequate, not too rich nutrition, and more physical activity in the poorer boys.

Food intake, energy expenditure, and habitual physical activity of nonindustrialized population groups were studied extensively (see Lange Andersen et al., 1978, for references). Calorie intakes are usually low (Table 2), but in several instances they are comparable with the 2,400−2,600 kcal/day (10.0−10.9 MJ/day) found by Durnin and Passmore (1967) and by Shock (1972) in men from industrialized counties who are engaged in sedentary work.

Physical fitness, expressed as maximum oxygen uptake, of nonindustrialized people is somewhat superior to that of industrialized

Table 2.   Examples of 24-hr caloric intake of adult inhabitants of simple hunting and nomadic communities

	24-hr caloric intake	
	(kcal)	(MJ)
Tropical and subtropical populations		
Kalahari bushmen	2,140	8.94
Indian tribes	1,860−3,100	7.77−12.96
Cook Island Maoris—men	1,840−2,200	7.69−9.20
—women	1,760−1,980	7.36−8.28
East Java villagers	1,000−1,500	4.18−6.27
Philippine villagers	1,670	6.98
Negev bedouins	1,360−2,650	5.68−11.08
New Guinea villagers—men	2,300	9.61
—women	1,700	7.11
Brazilian villagers	2,500	10.45
Ibo tribes, Nigeria	2,350	9.82
Baganda peasants, Uganda	2,000	8.36
Quechua Indians, Peru	2,500	10.45
Arctic and Subarctic populations		
Canadian Eskimo—men	2,097−2,860	8.76−11.95
—women	2,500	10.45
Alaskan Eskimo and Indians—men	1,500−2,650	6.27−11.08
Athabascan Indians—men	2,250	9.40
Lapps of Northern Norway—men	2,400	10.03
—women	1,800	7.52
Skolts of Northern Finland—men	2,200	9.20
—women	1,700	7.11

Caucasians (Table 3). Absence of overnutrition and a high level of habitual physical activity have often been thought to be responsible for the rarity of ischemic heart disease in the less affluent population groups of developing countries. However, transition from diets now characteristic of most of the developing countries to those more typical of the industrialized countries would imply a marked increase in the intake of animal fats and hence in saturated fatty acids, and in dietary cholesterol. Sucrose intake could also increase. If life styles as well as dietary patterns change, one might expect decreased physical activity and increased obesity. All these transformations would have to be viewed as increasing the risk of ischemic heart disease (Beaton and Bengoa, 1976).

Table 3. Maximum aerobic power in ml/min/kg of adult men of different societies

Society	Vo_2 max (ml/min/kg)
Nonindustrialized Arctic and Subarctic communities	
Igloolik Eskimos	58
Nomadic Lapps	54
Athabaskan Indians	49
Skolts (Northern Finland)	47
Wainwright Eskimos	45
Baffin Island Eskimos	44
Greenland Eskimos	41
Alucaluf Indians (Tierra del Fuego)	38
Nonindustrialized tropical and subtropical communities	
Masai, Tanzania	54
Pygmies, Zaire	48
Bushmen, Kalahari	47
Iutu, South Africa	45
Xhora, South Africa	45
Swazi, South Africa	45
Warao Indians, Venezuela	45
Basuto, South Africa	44
Bantu, Zaire	43
Pascuans, Easter Island	41
Venda, South Africa	40
Ethiopians	35
Industrialized "western" communities	
Norway	47
Canada	39
Czechoslovakia	36
Belgium	36
USA	36

CONCLUSIONS

Physical fitness, acquired in youth and maintained throughout life by means of an appropriate pattern of habitual physical activity, including sport, is thought to exert beneficial effects on the locomotor, the digestive, the respiratory, and the cardiovascular systems, as well as on cell metabolism and organ functions in general. There are also psychological benefits to be gained from leading a physically active life. There is a controversy over whether physical fitness really prolongs life, and many studies carried out on athletes have failed to show significant beneficial effects on longevity. It is not enough to have been an athlete in youth. Former athletes do not fare any better than the general population in terms of longevity and cardiovascular health, and there is no carry-over of the beneficial health effects of physical fitness several decades later.

Although no clear-cut proof that physical activity prevents cardio-vascular diseases and prolongs life is available, there is plenty of circumstantial evidence that regular physical activity is essential for optimal body function and health, and is of value in preventive and in rehabilitation cardiology. If everyday life and work are not very demanding physically, a prudent attitude is that some physical activity be included during leisure time to provide the body with the stimuli it needs to function at its best, limit the occurrence and severity of certain degenerative diseases, particularly ischemic heart disease, and improve the chances of satisfactory recovery should such diseases occur.

REFERENCES

Beaton, G. H., and Bengoa, J. M. (eds.). 1976. Nutrition in Preventive Medicine. World Health Organization, Geneva.

Durnin, J. V. G. A., and Passmore, R. 1967. Energy, Work, and Leisure. Heinemann, London.

Epstein, L., et al. 1976. Vigorous exercise in leisure time, coronary risk factors, and resting electrocardiogram in middle-aged male civil servants. Br. Heart J. 38: 403−409.

Fejfar, Z., and Masironi, R. 1970. Dietary factors and cardiovascular dis-eases—Epidemiological studies in man. In 3rd Int. Congr. Food Sci. and Technol., August 9−14, Institute Food Technologists, Chicago, Il. SOS/70 Proc., Washington, D.C.

Fletcher, G. F., and Cantwell, J. D. 1974. Exercise and Coronary Heart Disease. Charles C Thomas Publisher, Springfield, Il.

Froelicher, V. F., and Oberman, A. 1972. Analysis of epidemiologic studies of physical inactivity as risk factors for coronary artery disease. Progr. Cardiovasc. Dis. 15(1): 41−65.

Gottheiner, V. 1968. Long-range strenuous sports training for cardiac recondi-tioning and rehabilitation. Am. J. Cardiol. 22: 426−435.

Hickey, N., et al. 1975. Study of coronary risk factors related to physical activity in 15171 men. Br. Med. J. 30 Aug.: 507−509.

Hildes, J. A., et al. 1976. Chronic lung disease and cardiovascular conse-quences in Iglooligmiut. In R.J. Shephard and S. Itoh (eds.), Circumpolar Health, pp. 327−331. Univ. of Toronto Press, Toronto.

International Society of Cardiology. 1973. Myocardial infarction: How to prevent, how to rehabilitate.

Johnson, M. L., et al. 1956. Prevalence and incidence of obesity of a cross-section of elementary and secondary school children. Am. J. Clin. Nutr. 4: 231−238.

Kagan, A. R., et al. 1977. Atherosclerosis of the aorta and coronary arteries in five towns. Bull. World Health Org. 53 (5−6): 485−645.

Lange Andersen, K. 1973. The effect of altitude variation on the physical performance capacity during adolescence. In V. Seliger (ed.), Physical Fitness, pp. 34−46. Charles University, Prague.

Lange Andersen, K., and Elvis, A. 1956. The resting arterial blood pressure in athletes. Acta Med. Scand. 153: 367−371.

Lange Andersen, K., et al. 1978. Habitual physical activity and health. WHO Regional Publications European Series, World Health Organization Regional Office for Europe, Copenhagen.

Mann, G. V., et al. 1965. Physical fitness and immunity to heart disease in Masai. Lancet 2: 1308–1310.

Mayer, J., et al. 1956. Relation between caloric intake, body weight, and physical work. Am. J. Clin. Nutr. 4: 169–175.

Miller, G. J., and Miller, N. E. 1975. Plasma high-density lipoprotein concentration and development of ischemic heart disease. Lancet 1: 16.

Montoye, H. J., et al. 1972. Habitual physical activity and blood pressure. Med. Sci. Sports 4 (4): 175–181.

Montoye, H. J., et al. 1976. Habitual physical activity and serum lipids of males, age 16–64 in a total community. J. Chron. Dis. 29: 697–710.

Morris, J. N., et al. 1953. Coronary heart disease and physical activity of work. Lancet 2: 1053–1057.

Morris, J. N., et al. 1973. Vigorous exercise in leisure-time and the incidence of coronary heart disease. Lancet 1: 333–339.

Pařízková, J. 1974. Interrelationship between body size, body composition, and function. In A.F. Roche and F. Falkner (eds.), Nutrition and Malnutrition. Adv. Exp. Med. Biol. 49: 119–149, Plenum Press, New York.

Prior, I. A. M., et al. 1966. The health of two groups of Cook Island Maoris, Dept. of Health Special Rep. Series No. 26, Medical Res. Council of New Zealand, Wellington.

Pyörälä, K., et al. 1967. Cardiovascular studies on former athletes. Am. J. Cardiol. 20: 191–205.

Rissanen, V. 1976. Occupational physical activity and coronary heart disease. Adv. Cardiol. 18: 113–121. Karger, Basel.

Sarajas, H. S. S. 1976. Reaction patterns of blood platelets in exercise. Adv. Cardiol. 18: 176–195.

Sedov, K. R. 1976. Epidemiology of some non-infectious diseases in Eastern Siberia. In R.J. Shephard and S. Itoh (eds.), Circumpolar Health, pp. 269–274. University of Toronto Press, Toronto.

Shirai, I. 1975. Nutrition and physical fitness. In K. Asahina and R. Shigiya (eds.), Physiological Adaptability and Nutritional Status of the Japanese (B), pp. 100–107. JIBP Synthesis, Vol. 4, Japanese Int. Biol. Prog. University of Tokyo.

Shock, N. W. 1972. Energy metabolism, caloric intake, and physical activity in the ageing. In L.A. Carlson (ed.), Nutrition in Old Age, pp. 12–13. Swedish Nutr. Foundation Symposium No. 10, Uppsala.

Skinner, J. S., et al. 1964. Effects of a programme of endurance exercises on physical work. Am. J. Cardiol. 14: 747–751.

Stefanik, P. A., et al. 1959. Caloric intake in relation to energy output of obese and nonobese adolescent boys. Am. J. Clin. Nutr. 7: 55–62.

Suzuki, S. 1975. Experimental studies on the interrelationship among nutrition, physical exercise and health components. In K. Asahina and R. Shigiya (eds.), Physiological Adaptability and Nutritional Status of the Japanese (B), pp. 83–94. JIBP Synthesis, Vol. 4, Japanese International Biological Programme, University of Tokyo Press.

Watt, E. W., et al. 1976a. Dietary intake and coronary risk factors in Peruvian Quechua Indians. J. Am. Diet. Ass. 68: 535–537.

Watt, E. W., et al. 1976b. Effect of dietary control and exercise training on daily food intake and serum lipids in postmyocardial infarction patients. Am. J. Clin. Nutr. 29: 900–904.

WHO. 1969. International work in cardiovascular diseases, 1959–1969. World Health Organization, Geneva.

WHO. 1976. Myocardial Infarction Community Registers. Public Health in Europe No. 5. World Health Organization, Regional Office for Europe, Copenhagen.

Interrelationships Between Nutrition, Physical Activity, and Cardiovascular Health

Z. Fejfar

The relationship between nutrition and physical activity is dealt with in this chapter from the experimental, physiological, and epidemiological points of view. The expected positive correlation between these variables appears within fairly wide limits. However, the relationship becomes negative at the higher levels of nutritional status in the now so-called developed countries and in the well-to-do social groups elsewhere, where abundant nutrition is accompanied by a relatively low level of physical activity. Obesity can be considered an expression of increasing wealth and of less improved or impaired health in these communities.

Qualitative changes in nutrition are known to influence mental and physical status, and experimental studies by Suzuki et al. (this volume) indicate clearly that the voluntary physical activity was higher in rats nourished predominantly with proteins and fat as compared with those on a high carbohydrate diet. There seems to be no doubt concerning the importance of a supply of glucose to replenish the liver stores, in long and demanding exercise. On the other hand, opinion differs as to the optimal requirement of proteins for physical activity and fitness in human populations.

As far as the relationship between nutrition and fitness is concerned, the correlation is poor within a broad range of food intakes. Physical fitness is defined as the ability to perform muscular work satisfactorily under specified conditions (WHO, 1968). It may be assessed by the magnitude, duration, and the type of maximum exercise that a subject can perform, by the relationship between the level of submaximal exercise and the body response to it, by the rapidity of recovery of the cardiorespiratory system from such exercise, and by the degree of fatigue if engaged in prolonged activity.

As for the association between physical activity (be it static or dynamic work) and fitness, several symposia and publications exist that provide fairly complete information. The correlation between fitness for a given type of physical activity and the ability to perform maximal short-lasting effort and the habitual physical activity is rather complex, and is dealt with later.

If one reviews available information on nutritional changes associated with economic growth, the picture seems clear when comparing data from different countries as well as when comparing the more fortunate with the less well-to-do groups within a given country. The higher the per capita national product, the higher the percentage of fat, and the greater the amount of animal, saturated, and separated vegetable fat, the higher the intake of pure carbohydrate and the greater the decrease in starch. The total protein consumption does not change much, but a greater percentage comes from the animal compared to vegetable and fish protein (FAO, 1969; Masironi, 1970).

It is well known, of course, that high calorie intake with a great percentage of fat is associated with hyperlipidemia, which in turn is related to the frequency of ischemic heart disease (IHD). In fact, in populations with low blood lipids (cholesterol and triglycerides, and essentially in those where the mean serum cholesterol levels are below 200 mg/dl (Fejfar and Masironi, 1971), IHD is rare, and if it does occur it is usually not related to the coronary atherosclerosis.

Although the increase in caloric intake from birth is manifested in greater physical growth, this does not imply greater physical activity, greater performance, or better health. It is now well known that "too much may not be so good." This applies in particular to the nutritional habits in early childhood.

It has also been known for a long time that industrial development is characterized by diminishing hard physical labor, by quantitative and qualitative changes in the diet, by increased cigarette smoking, and by rising mental stress, which is partly related to the increasing speed in most of our daily activities. The interest in sport has increased more or less hand in hand with the industrialization process, and one wonders to what extent it might be an expression of the subconscious compensatory efforts for our sedentary life.

The great emphasis and high priority on the top athletes (who resemble more and more the Roman Empire gladiators) who are officially supported in many countries of the world has some justification in providing an example for the youth.

However, it contrasts markedly with facilities that inadequately satisfy for the masses the basic need for pleasure in physical activity, not to mention the positive influence on health such activity provides.

The result has been the development in the 1950s and 1960s of a young and middle-age population with low levels of physical activity, increased body weight, and increased aggressiveness as shown in daily life, and which is quite evident when watching sport competitions.

As for the relationship of physical activity to cardiovascular health and disease, the enormous amount of literature published since the time when Morris et al. (1953) outlined the hypothesis about the beneficial effect of physical activity for cardiovascular health does not contain a great deal of well-documented data. The reasons for this are many. We can measure, with considerable accuracy, physical performance and the energy expenditure during a short period of activity. On the other hand, great problems arise when one attempts to estimate habitual activity during work and during leisure.

Let us start with the assumption that a change in the habitual physical activity of populations, coupled with other behavior changes—smoking habits, abundant nutrition, and lack of mental adaptation to the man-made environment, for example—may be contributing factors to the development of premature ischemic heart disease (IHD). In order to prove this, one should separate the activity from the other factors mentioned and prove to what extent they are independent, additive, or compensatory. For all this, of course, one must have a reliable method for the measurement of all parameters. It is perhaps surprising for the layman, but nevertheless useful to reemphasize, that there are great difficulties in measuring *habitual* diet and *habitual physical* activity, the two basic features of daily life. Moreover, even greater problems are encountered when one attempts to measure the effect of mental stimuli on the organism.

Habitual physical activity obviously varies with age and sex. It varies in most of us from day to day, from season to season. The diminishing requirements for physical activity in most jobs shift the emphasis toward the physical work load during leisure. The direct measurement of the habitual physical activity is at present difficult, time consuming, and arduous (WHO, 1969). The diary technique (timing and recording of activity by the subject) is suitable for large groups, providing that the reliability can be tested in repeated observations.

A number of indirect techniques exist in which one measures the response of the organism to various stimuli (physical, mental, environmental). Assessment of the energy consumption from estimation of the O_2 or from the dietary intake are difficult for long-term measurement in population groups. For determination of the cardiovascular and metabolic responses to activity, recording of the heart rate seems most suitable, although the changes are influenced by mental stimuli, heat, and other environmental stimuli.

Direct measurements can be recorded on a small number of the subjects and the indirect determinations, either actual description of the activity in the diaries and/or the measurement of the heart frequency, seem more practical, but until now results are available from only a few studies.

The technique described by Masironi and Mansourian (1974) enables one to measure R-R intervals and thus, to record the heart function over a chosen time period (for several hours) and also the distribution of the heart rates into eight frequency classes. This, together with a simple diary, should give a good picture of the day and night physical activity of the individual.

Long-term follow-up of active sportsmen regarding their cardiovascular health also has a number of biases. Some are inherent in the difficulties associated with the diagnosis of the coronary sclerosis in man without symptoms and signs, and others in the complex nature of IHD, in which the development is related to several environmental influences, of which physical activity and inactivity are only two of many. Furthermore, it is well known that a number of top competitors alter their way of life soon after retiring from active competition. In such situations, it is difficult to relate any changes in their health status 5–10 years later to their previous activity. This is one of the reasons why the proposal to keep medical records of the active Olympic Games participants—the so-called Olympic Medical Archives—was unrealistic. Direct proof from longitudinal studies showing that physical activity prolongs life or prevents the development or even prognosis of IHD is lacking.

It has been repeatedly demonstrated that physical activity during convalescence from acute myocardial infarction (AMI) does not make victims worse and does not increase the frequency of complications. Most of these individuals feel better off and enjoy life more than the inactive ones.

Observation of convalescents from AMI did not disclose harmful effects of physical activity, even in subjects with hemodynamic signs of an insufficient ventricle (Ressl et al., 1975). Subjects can improve their physical fitness, and the present trends seem to be toward becoming more active in spite of the lack of knowledge about the long-term effects of physical activity on mortality and morbidity.

An investigation to prove this would be difficult to plan. One cannot "blindly" observe active and inactive populations. The WHO group of experts in Moscow in 1972 succeeded in planning and initiating a cooperative study with the aim to demonstrate the effect of an organized physical activity program as a secondary preventive measure in randomly selected patients who were physically active, and in inactive groups of patients who recovered from AMI. The study is under-way in a number of European centers and is progressing well.

In observational studies in which the physical activity at work and during leisure has been assessed, those more physically active suffered less from IHD than the less active groups (Fox, 1972), but Chapman et al.'s study (1957) on longshoremen in Los Angeles seems to be an exception to the rule.

The only prospective primary prevention study designed to eluci-date the relation between physical activity during leisure time and fu-ture cardiovascular disease is that by Morris et al. (1973). Approxi-mately 17,000 male, middle-age civil servants in the United Kingdom were asked during 1968–1970 to record on Monday morning their lei-sure time activity during the preceeding Friday and Saturday. It has been shown that those reporting *vigorous* exercise had a lower rate of IHD (both mortality and morbidity) than the well-matched group of less active subjects. Vigorous exercise was defined as that requiring a peak energy expenditure of 7.5kcal/min (31.5 J/min/liter). This energy expenditure in specified exercise continued for at least 5 min, and the "heavy work" continued for more than 30 min, or totaled at least 1 hr over the two days.

Examples of vigorous exercise in leisure time (adapted from Mor-ris et al., 1973) are displayed below:

Vigorous exercise	Heavy work
Swimming	"Do it yourself" activities
Hill climbing	such as
Dancing (specified exercise)	Gardening
Morning exercises (Jogging)	Digging
Brisk walking	Felling trees
Running	Clearing scrub
Cycling (specified exercise)	Building in stone or concrete
Climbing up stairs	Moving heavy objects
450 + daily	

A sample of 600 of the original population was asked in 1971 to complete an additional questionnaire consisting of medical, social, and smoking histories. These men were given an electrocardiogram at rest, and blood pressure and blood cholesterol were measured. There were 509 subjects who completed these procedures, which was a 77% re-sponse rate. Of this sample, 125 individuals reported previously vigor-ous exercise. They differed from others in that they showed fewer abnormalities on the ECG (Minnesota code criteria), indicating possi-ble myocardial ischemia, ectopic beats, or sinus tachycardia (Epstein et al., 1976).

The question is not whether to exercise, but when to do it and to what extent.

Physical activity has been discussed so far from the epidemiological aspect. There are considerable data indicating the harmful effects of very strenuous efforts, the degree and circumstances of which point to great emotional strain (fear, anxiety). In such situations physical effort is by necessity often overshadowed by an acute catecholamine storm, sudden exhaustion, circulatory collapse, signs of acute myocardial ischemia, or even sudden death. The exceptional physical effort and its harmful consequences is contrasted to physical inactivity, a much more common danger, particularly when coupled with psychic strain and abundant nutrition.

PERSPECTIVES

The trend of diminishing physical activity at work and better transportation facilities has not been compensated for by additional physical effort during leisure time in many advanced communities. This, as well as steadily abundant nutrition, is manifested in a sizable percentage of overweight adults. It also seems easier to lose extra weight by increasing physical activity than by reducing the total calorie intake and/or by using particular diets (see Šonka, Apfelbaum et al., this volume).

Fuel supply and physical activity are both basic manifestations of life, yet we not only have problems concerning how to measure them, but controversies regarding the amount and type needed for optimum health.

We cannot neglect observations in the study of the survival of previously active sportsmen, either. Their mortality from cardiovascular diseases is similar to that of the normal population, and in some studies there are indications of the increased CVD mortality in former athletes (Polednak and Damon, 1970; Schmid, Hornof, and Král, 1975).

On the other hand, there has been a slow but steady decline in the mortality from these conditions during the past few years in America (HEW News, 1975). To what extent this might be related to a rather rapid reorientation of a population toward increasing physical activity in recent years, if indeed this is correct, is a speculation that should be answered within a few years.

The simple equation, energy balance equals energy expenditure and dietary intake, becomes a rather complicated matter in a life situation, where many factors—age, environmental changes, and disease—may interact or intervene.

Observations on subjects born and living at high altitudes (over 3,000 m) show a physical performance similar to that of lowlanders.

This is so despite the fact that the coronary blood flow is not elevated (Grover and Alexander, 1972; Moret, 1972), and thus the amount of oxygen delivered to the heart muscle cells is decreased. The preference for lactate utilization by the heart muscle cannot fully explain the normal cardiac work efficiency. It has been concluded that adaptation to this environmental situation must be at the level of the heart muscle cell, in the mitochondrial enzyme structure and function.

There is general agreement and considerable data on circulatory, respiratory, and metabolic adaptation by training. This is in contrast, however, to the paucity of information on the duration of the training effect.

Data by Robinson et al. (1972) on the effects of training on physiological aging of well-trained subjects, re-studied 21 and 31 years later, did not show a persistent effect from the past vigorous training at the age of 20. Their work capacity and Vo_2 max were similar to those of other men of a like age. During the 30 years, these subjects gained on the average about 10 kg in weight, and their body fat increased by more than 20%. The data confirm previous observations that training in young age does not increase aerobic capacity in middle-age men who do not continue with the training. In this respect, interesting experimental data by Pařízková (1975, 1977) show that the offspring of rat mothers exercised daily throughout pregnancy, and starting within 2−3 days after mating, had heavier hearts with a greater number of fibers and a particularly greater number of capillaries, so that the capillary/ fiber ratio was higher.

Although we do not know how long such training effect would persist after birth, one can speculate that, given the proper high protein diet (see Suzuki et al., this volume), the animals might continue to be more physically active, and hence would develop a higher work capacity. It is, of course, difficult to extrapolate from rat to man. Nevertheless, one can at least consider that under normal circumstances, metabolic, circulatory, and respiratory adjustments to increased physical activity since childhood will have a lasting effect on the organism. These effects might be hidden during periods of inactivity, but they are not lost. Therefore, those who have been physically active since childhood more easily recover these effects than those who have not always been active. In this respect, Pařízková (1975, 1977) provides a fascinating model for further research.

Metabolic and hormonal stimuli of the fetus and dynamic exercise starting early after birth increases activity of the lipid metabolism (Pařízková, 1977). Can this be considered as a model for humans? There are communities with frequent coronary atherosclerosis, with marked rise of blood cholesterol levels within 2−3 years after birth.

The interest for studying atherogenesis in early childhood has been gaining more and more attention in recent years and we are looking forward now to facts (Uppal and Arntzenius, 1974; WHO, 1974). We cannot expect definitive answers from large scale preventive programs on the effects of physical activity and inactivity on atherogenesis and on the development of IHD (Fejfar, 1975).

There is no easy way to demonstrate the beneficial influence of moderate physical activity throughout life on health. There is an urgent need to know more about the regulatory mechanisms in man during the aging processes from the metabolic, circulatory, and respiratory point of view. This information must be oriented toward physical and mental effort. Health is defined as physical, mental, and also social well-being. The factual knowledge and objective measurements of psychic effect on health are negligible, although experience and observation indicate an increasing and seemingly often decisive influence of psychic stress.

REFERENCES

Chapman, J. M., Goerke, L. S., Dixon, W., Loveland, D. B., and Philips, E. 1957. The clinical status of a population group in Los Angeles under observation for two to three years. Am. J. Public Health. 47: 33.

The Effect of Rehabilitation and Secondary Prevention in Patients with Acute Myocardial Infarction. 1976. Report on working group. September 10–13, 1975, Opatija. EURO, ICP/CVI/005 (10).

Epstein, L., Miller, G. J., Stitt, F. W., and Morris, J. N. 1976. Vigorous exercise in leisure time, coronary risk-factors, and resting electrocardiogram in middle-aged male civil servants. Brit. Heart J. 38: 403–409.

Evaluation of Comprehensive Rehabilitative and Preventive Programs for Patients after Acute Myocardial Infarction. Report on two working groups. 1973. October 4–7, 1971, Prague; November 27–30, 1972, Moscow. EURO, 8206/8.

Fejfar, Z. 1975. Prevention against ischaemic heart disease: A critical review. In M. F. Oliver (ed.), Modern Trends in Cardiology. Butterworths, London and Boston.

Fejfar, Z., and Masironi, R. 1971. Dietary factors and cardiovascular diseases—Epidemiological studies in man. In Proceedings of the 3rd International Congress of Food Science and Technology, August 9–14, 1970, Washington, D. C.

FAO. 1969. Provisional indicative world plan for agricultural development: A synthesis and analysis of factors relevant to world, regional and national agricultural development. FAO 2: C69/4.

Fox, S. M. III. 1972. Physical activity and coronary heart disease. In Edward K. Chung (ed.), Controversy in Cardiology: The Practical Clinical Approach, pp. 201–219. Springer-Verlag, New York.

HEW News. 1975.

Grover, R. F., and Alexander, J. K. 1972. Cardiac performance and coronary circulation of man in chronic hypoxia. Cardiology 56: 197–206.

Masironi, R. 1970. Dietary factors and coronary heart disease. Bull. World Health Org. 42: 103–114.

Masironi, R., and Mansourian, P. 1974. Determination of habitual physical activity by means of a portable R-R interval distribution recorder. Bull. World Health Org. 51: 291–298.

Moret, P. 1972. Myocardial changes in chronic hypoxia. Cardiology 56: 161–192.

Morris, J. N., Chave, S. P. W., Adam, C., Sirey, E., Epstein, L., and Sheehan, D. J. 1973. Vigorous exercise in leisure-time and the incidence of coronary heart disease. Lancet 1: 333.

Morris, J. N., Heady, J. A., Raffle, P. A. B., Roberts, C. G., and Parks, J. W. 1953. Coronary heart disease and physical activity of work. Lancet 2: 1053.

Pařízková, J. 1975. Body Fat and Physical Fitness. Martinus Nijhoff B.V./ Medical Division, The Hague.

Pařízková, J. 1977. Impact of daily work-load during pregnancy on the microstructure of the rat heart in male offspring. Europ. J. Appl. Physiol. 34: 323.

Polednak, A. P., and Damon, A. 1970. College athletics, longevity, and cause of death. Hum. Biol. 42: 28.

Ressl, J., Jandová, R., Stolz, I., and Widimský, J. 1975. Effects of physical training on central haemodynamics and working capacity in myocardial infarction. Cor Vasa 17 (4): 241–253.

Robinson, S. D. B., Dill, R., Robinson, R. D., Wagner, J. A., and Tzankoff, S. P. 1972. Training and physiological aging in man. Fed. Proc. 32: 1628–1634.

Schmid, L., Hornof, Z., and Král, J. 1975. Náhlé úmrté při afekcich kardiovaskulárního aparátu při sportu. In Náhlé Úmrtia, p. 91. Martin.

Uppal, S. C., and Arntzenius, A. C. 1974. Westland school children survey. A preliminary report on risk factors for CHD. Heart Bull. 5: 95–98.

WHO. 1974. Study of atherosclerosis precursors in children. Report of WHO consultation on Prevention of adult Cardiovascular diseases in childhood, February 4–6, Geneva. CVD/74.4.

WHO. 1968. Exercise tests in relation to cardiovascular function. Report of a meeting. Technical Report Serv. 388.

Summary Remarks

Summary Remarks

J. Pařízková

The presented selection of contributions on the interrelationships between nutrition, physical activity, and fitness has given some idea about the present status of research on this topic and its importance in connection with many other theoretical, clinical, and practical aspects. These problems deservedly are the center of interest in many laboratories.

The evaluation of the nutritional status of the organism resulting from lifelong energy intake and/or balance cannot be conceived as merely the absence of deficiency symptoms. There is a need, from the point of view of desirable health status, to go further and define in greater detail all qualities of the organism, including its functional capacity and its relationship to all factors that can influence it. Nutrition is obviously one of the most fundamental factors.

Achievement of the optimal functional capacity together with good somatic development is of basic importance to the desirable growth and development of the child during various stages of ontogeny and, above all, to the health prognosis. A high level of functional capacity, the definition of which varies according to activity, is important in adult age for economic production, which influences the economic level of the family. This is essential first of all for developing countries. This aspect is desirable for both men and women; moreover, women need an optimal functional capacity for childbearing and producing healthy and fit offspring. Longevity and good health, with a high level of productivity until advanced age, is another important aim when considering the desirable relationship between nutrition and performance capacity. Last, but not least, the interest in champion sport and successful representation of the country in top international competition has become a topic of keen interest in both developed and developing countries.

Adequate nutrition plays an essential role in all aspects of life. The kinds of diets maintained over long periods contribute to the creation of either good or bad predispositions for physical performance. Minor deficiencies, encountered often even in affluent societies and not necessarily caused by lack of food, interfere seriously with higher fitness and the expected level of functional capacity. There is no need to mention that starvation and hunger are contradictory to good performance capacity. Nevertheless, smaller body size resulting from chronically limited energy intake can often be associated with a satisfactory level of performance capacity for selected tasks and very good health. An example of this is the specialized athlete (e.g., gymnasts), in whose sport discipline the higher or even "normal" body weight and fatness interferes with good performance, and a carefully monitored and reduced energy intake is required.

Interindividual variations ("nutritional individuality") were related to a certain metabolic pattern and motor activity type, and demonstrated that the same nutrition—poor or good—can have a specific effect in individual subjects. Basic knowledge about the elementary mechanisms directing the metabolic processes in the organism concerning basic nutrients, water, electrolytes, etc. and resulting, inter alia, also in a different level of physical fitness and performance capacity, has to be gained in experimental studies in both human subjects as well as in laboratory animals. On the other hand, epidemiological and ecological, as well as clinical, studies are indispensable for the comprehensive understanding of the exact role of nutrition in creating the optimal fitness and performance capacity. There are still possibilities concerning how to enhance, modify, and economize the role of nutrition to achieve better results. This especially concerns problems of health and longevity.

There exist mainly two extreme deviations of the nutritional status: undernourished or malnourished subjects from the developing countries, who mostly (but not necessarily) display a low level of performance capacity; and overnourished hypokinetic subjects from developed countries, who are suffering more and more from so-called "diseases of civilization," and who have a low level of overall physical fitness that has deteriorated for quite opposite reasons. It would be desirable on the basis of all accessible data to define as precisely as possible the optimal (but not maximal) diet for the typical man both from the quantitative and qualitative point of view with regard to his enormously differentiated needs and specific features in various parts of the world. This ought to result in the ideal level of functional capacity in both the physical and mental sphere and finally be reflected in all possible areas of human activities. Until now, we have very few reasons to feel satisfied in this respect.